POWERSCULPT
FOR WOMEN

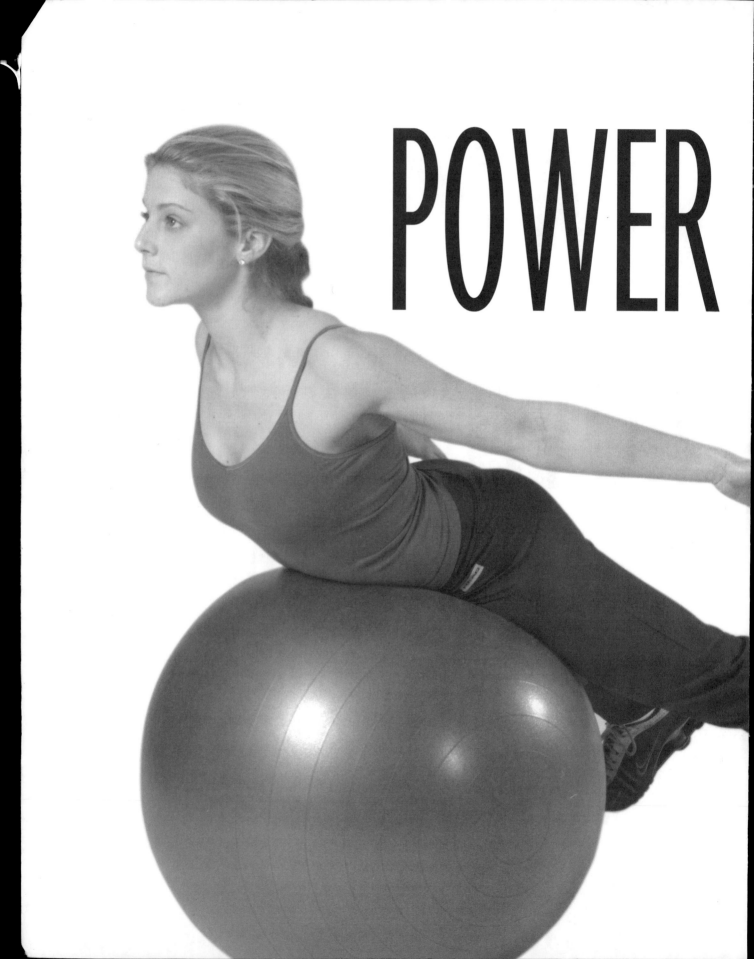

POWER

SCULPT FOR WOMEN

The Complete
Body Sculpting &
Weight Training Workout
Using the Exercise Ball

By PAUL FREDIANI

PHOTOGRAPHS *by* PETER FIELD PECK

healthylivingbooks
NEW YORK · LONDON

Text ©2005 Paul Frediani
Photographs ©2005 Hatherleigh Press

healthyliving**books**
Published by Hatherleigh Press
5-22 46th Avenue, Suite 200
Long Island City, NY 11101
Visit our Web site:
www.healthylivingbooks.com

Frediani, Paul, 1952-
  Powersculpt for women : the complete body sculpting & weight training workout using the exercise ball / by Paul Frediani ; photographs by Peter Field Peck.
     p. cm.
   ISBN 1-57826-182-1
   1. Exercise for women. 2. Weight training for women. 3. Swiss exercise balls. I. Title.
   GV482.F74 2004
   613.7'045--dc22

                                    2004023783

Seek the advice of your physician before starting any physical fitness program.

HEALTHY LIVING BOOKS are available for bulk purchase, special promotions, and premiums. For information on reselling and special purchase opportunities, please call us at 1-800-528-2550 and ask the the Special Sales Manager.

Cover and interior design by Corin Hirsch and Deborah Miller

10 9 8 7 6 5 4 3 2 1
Printed in Canada

Acknowledgments

Special thanks to my publisher Andrew Flach, my editor Lori Baird, designer Corin Hirsch, photographer Peter Peck, and our models, Renata Darlen and Cindy Sherwin. All made working on *PowerSculpt* a pleasure. I'd also like to thank the educators in the fitness industry that have elevated the level and knowledge of fitness professionals. Special thanks to Paul Chek and Juan Carlos Santana for their inspiring workshops and seminars.

To my clients for their support and trust.

To Paul West, Director of The United States Surfing Federation, for giving the opportunity of training team members.

Most of all to my family and friends who always believed in me.

Table of
Conte

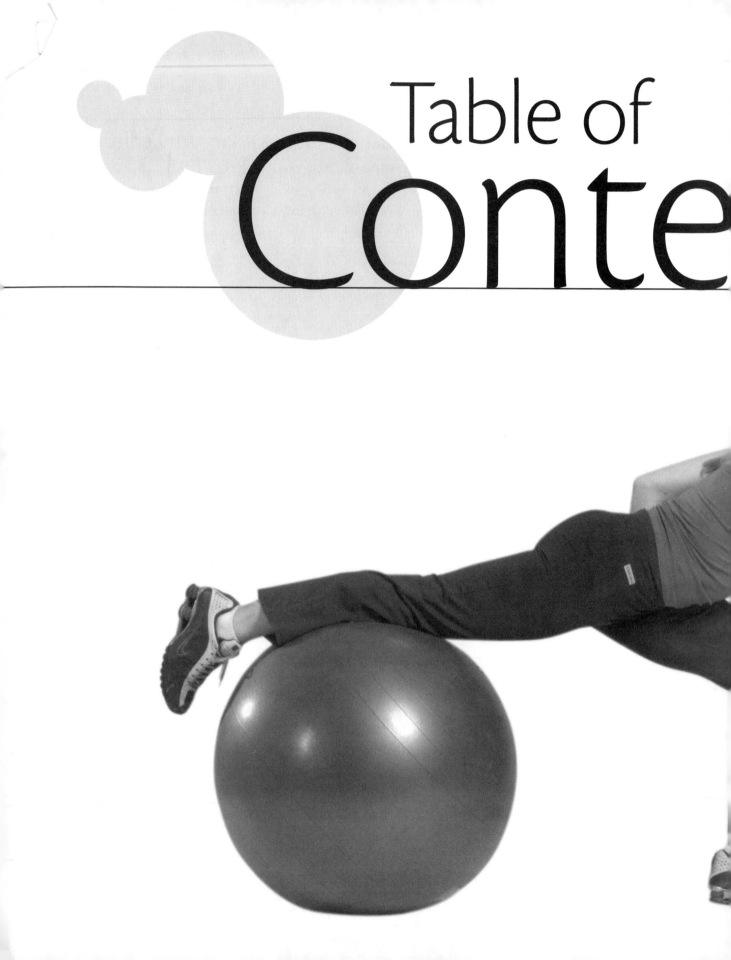

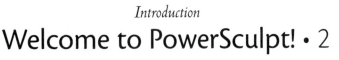

Introduction

Welcome to PowerSculpt! • 2

Connecting with Your Core • The PowerSculpt Difference
About the PowerSculpt Workouts

Chapter 1

The Power of Proper Posture • 8

Chapter 2

Getting Acquainted with the Fitness Ball • 12

Fitness Ball Basics • Balance and Stability on the Ball

Chapter 3

The PowerSculpt 10-Minute Warm-Up • 26

Chapter 4

The PowerSculpt Moves • 38

Chest • Back • Shoulders • Arms • Abs • Legs • Glutes • Neck

Chapter 5

PowerSculpt Flexibility Training • 114

Chapter 6

PowerSculpt Balance • 124

Chapter 7

The PowerSculpt Workouts • 134

Welcome to PowerS

Several years ago, an associate introduced me to the fitness ball. I struggled with every exercise she showed me. Within minutes, beads of sweat poured down my face; it felt as if I was wrestling an alligator.

I'm quite fit, so I was surprised by my inability to perform even simple exercises on the ball while maintaining my balance.

Working on the ball that day was a humbling experience, but I had a feeling that fitness ball training could open a whole new world of excellent and exciting possibilities for physical conditioning.

That first experience led me to Paul Chek and Juan Carlos Santana, two of the nation's leading fitness experts and educators, and two of the best sources of fitness ball training available. Their courses were priceless to me.

I began a daily regimen of working out on the ball. After I developed sufficient skill and knowledge, I began sharing what I had learned about the ball with my clients, some of whom achieved staggering accomplishments. Take, for example, a client I'll call Joan. At sixty, she had terrible balance problems, and within a year had broken an ankle and finger in separate falls. She couldn't even balance on one foot. Six month after starting work on the fitness ball, she could kneel on it and perform shoulder presses!

Another client, Maria, hadn't been able to do just one push-up with her knees off the floor.

culpt

A couple of months after incorporating fitness ball training into her workouts, she was cranking off ten pushups. Charlie sent me a bottle of expensive wine after his back pain was alleviated by the few simple ball warm-ups I suggested.

Monica was getting married and wanted to drop eight pounds in two months. An excellent athlete in superior shape, she had succeeded in everything from swimming to running to gymnastics. But she was also getting bored with her training routine and needed a boost to her motivation.

I introduced her to the fitness ball and she was immediately challenged and stimulated. Monica lost those eight pounds, got into even better shape, relieved her boredom, and got completely hooked on fitness ball training!

Sure, the evidence was anecdotal, but it proved even to someone as thick-headed as me the value of fitness ball training. I didn't have to wait for the scientific research to catch up to what I saw with my own eyes.

With this newly found enthusiasm and armed with a couple of dozen fitness balls, I designed a group fitness class and launched it at The Hamptons Boot Camp, a series of fitness classes I taught in Amagansett, New York, a few years back. The fitness ball class quickly became the most popular one offered. If fitness ball training received such a positive response and produced such wonderful results for the average person, I thought, how would it work for elite athletes?

I got my opportunity to find out when I was invited to travel with and train members of the United States Surfing Federation during a competition in the Dominican Republic. It was a richly rewarding experience. Working with these amazing athletes further expanded my knowledge and experience with the ball. I challenged them to highly complex movements and they took to the training like fish to water. Surfers love exercises that stimulate and challenge their balance systems. And though they were quite proficient at many of the advanced exercises, I was surprised at how they struggled with some of the basic stretches. It was further evidence that the repetitive movements required by sports can create imbalances in the body. If those imbalances are not checked, poor postural habits and injuries can result.

It was rewarding to hear those surfers acknowledge how fitness ball training enhanced their performance in the sport they love, and I'm sure many of them will be traveling with their fitness balls in tow.

Birth of the Ball

The fitness ball—also known as the Swiss ball, physio ball, or stability ball—was invented in the mid-nineteen sixties by an Italian toy manufacturer. It was first used in physical rehabilitation by Swiss spinal rehab specialist, Dr. Susan Klein-Vogelbach, who used the ball to help patients with orthopedic and other medical problems.

Connecting with Your Core

Core is a popular buzzword in fitness training these days. But what exactly is the core and why is it so important? Like the steel cables of a bridge, your core is the foundation and support system of your body. It stabilizes your spine and connects your upper and lower extremities. It is the central source of power and is essential for efficient movement. Furthermore, your core is your center of gravity, playing an essential role in helping you maintain balance and equilibrium. In short, a strong and stable core is crucial to optimum health and movement—whether you're hanging ten on your surfboard or carrying your groceries from the store and stepping off the curb.

Technically speaking, the core musculature includes your spine, your pelvic and shoulder girdles, and the muscles that act on these bony structures (back and hip muscles).

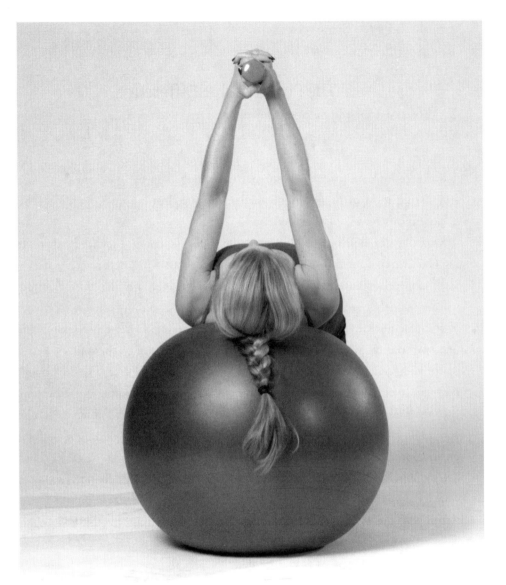

The Ball Today

These days, fitness ball training is being integrated with yoga, Pilates, pre- and postnatal exercise, senior exercise regimens, everyday flexibility, and functional training.

Working on the fitness ball not only helps develop the strength of your core muscles, but, because the ball is unstable, training on it also strengthens your stabilizing muscles. Those muscles are found at major joints and around your spine, hips, and shoulders. Most people don't train their stabilizing muscles, concentrating instead on the so-called major muscle groups of the chest, back, shoulders, hamstrings, quadriceps, biceps, and triceps. For those muscle groups to work together, create explosive movements, and lessen the possibility of injury, the smaller stabilizing muscles must be trained and well conditioned, too. Training on

Change is Good

If you never change your exercise routines, you'll never change your body. That's because over time your body adapts to the same routine. If you want to become stronger and more fit, then you must constantly change your workouts. Changing the speed, intensity, and stability of an exercise will do just that. And the fitness ball is the only piece of equipment that will allow you to do that.

the ball also strengthens your joints, and strong joints allow your body to move more powerfully, with more fluidity, and with less chance of injury.

The PowerSculpt Difference

Tired of the same old exercise routine: ten reps, wait, and do it again; waiting in line at the gym to use the new machine—that turns out to be as useless as the old machine?

If you're looking for a workout that will charge you up, give you fast results, is stimulating and fun, then look no further, because I promise you that PowerSculpt is like no other you've ever experienced.

Regardless of how old you are, what condition you're in, or what kinds of training you're accustomed to, the PowerSculpt Workout will get you to the next level, safely and progressively. It's not an easy workout; even a well-conditioned athlete will most likely need to start at the beginning levels, so don't get down on yourself if you tire quickly. Those twenty to thirty minutes of training per session for the first two to three weeks will be challenging. Why? Because of the way the ball stimulates your central nervous system and the synergistic kinesiology of fitness ball training. In other words, when you do the PowerSculpt Workout, you're bringing all your muscles to the party. You may be doing a chest exercise, but at the same time you'll be working your lower back, hips, butt, and legs. Or you might be focusing on an abdominal exercise and the same time working your chest, shoulders, and hip flexors. And if that's not enough, you will simultaneously be required to maintain your balance and posture.

You see, the PowerSculpt Workout doesn't isolate muscles the way those big clunky machines at the gym do. Muscle isolation is fine if you're a body builder, but most of the rest of us want a body that's lean, flexible, able to react quickly and fluidly, and works as a whole unit. Let's say you have to push a really heavy shopping cart, for example. It's not just your chest muscles that are doing the work. Your chest will work with your back, abs, legs, and myriad other muscles to create the power and movement you need. At the same time you need to maintain your balance to get proper leverage. There are no machines in the gym that will teach you how to do that. PowerSculpt does.

PowerSculpt will develop your strength through stability and balance. Your posture will change, you will become more poised, your flexibility will increase, and you'll lose inches, because of greater caloric burn resulting from the recruitment of more muscles. As your strength and balance increase, so will your level of training. You'll be able to chart your progress and and execute movements you never thought possible. After awhile, what you once considered a workout will be a warm-up. If you're looking to burn fat and tone your body, PowerSculpt is the road map that will get you there.

About the PowerSculpt Workouts

In the pages that follow, you'll learn everything you need to know about working out with the fitness ball. You'll start with balance and stability exercises, which are important because they help you identify your starting level.

After that you'll move on to the PowerSculpt 10-Minute Warm-Up. Do those exercises in sequence as a prelude to the more challenging workouts to come.

Chapter 4 is where you'll learn all the PowerSculpt moves. These exercises will challenge your stability, work your core, and strengthen and sculpt your whole body. They are also the exercises you'll use for the PowerSculpt Workouts.

In chapters 5 and 6, I acquaint you with some moves and poses designed especially to enhance your flexibility and balance.

Chapter 7 is where it all comes together in the PowerSculpt Workout, a progressive 12-week body sculpting plan. It couldn't be simpler: One hour a day, three days a week for 12 weeks. But I don't just throw you on the ball and wish you luck. My workouts guide you from the very beginning (Stage 1: Stability and Foundations) to an advanced body sculpting workout (Stage 4: Power).

I saved the best workout for last. It's the PowerSculpt Body Blast Circuit Workout. It's just one day a week for 10 weeks. That may sound too easy, but don't be fooled—there's a reason for six rest days every week!

So again, welcome to PowerSculpt. With the ball and this book, I guarantee you a workout like you've never seen!

Chapter 1

The Power of Proper Posture

Good posture is essential for good balance and energy. Almost every popular form of exercise—Feldenkrais®, Pilates, yoga—is based on achieving proper posture. In fact, Dr. Feldenkrais said, "Posture is where movement begins and ends."

Consider a 140-pound woman. Her head weighs about eleven pounds. If she slouches enough to shift her head forward about 3 1/2 inches, her head would feel like 15 1/2 pounds. If she continued to slouch forward from her waist and trunk by 7.6 degrees, the combined weight of her head and torso would seem like 138 pounds! Think about how exhausting it would be to carry around all that extra weight. Poor posture accelerates wear and tear on the body's joints and is a fast track to overuse injuries and arthritis. It can affect our ability to breathe properly, perform sports and everyday activities, and it most definitely affects how we look and feel about ourselves.

We must be aware of our posture everyday, not only when we exercise. But what is good posture? Chances are your posture isn't perfect. Tightness in one set of muscles and weakness in others can certainly affect your ability to stand up straight. Playing sports that require repetitive movements and small tasks you perform in your everyday life can have adverse effects on your posture. When you sit at your desk do you cross your legs? When standing, do you always lean on your dominant leg? Do you carry a purse or pack over one shoulder? Poor habits created over years take constant positive reeducation.

If you begin PowerSculpt with poor posture (we all have it to some degree) you need to pay close attention to your form while training. The good news is that awareness is the first step toward improvement and PowerSculpt will strengthen and stretch the muscles needed for better posture. Some of my clients have achieved positive postural changes in a matter of months. Funny thing is they were constantly being told how wonderful they looked and asked how much weight they had lost, when all they really did was improve their posture.

Proper Posture for PowerSculpt

How important is posture when it comes to PowerSculpt? Well, it governs whether or not you will be able to progress to more advanced exercises and avoid injury. If you try to advance through the exercises too quickly, you not only risk injuring yourself, but you also reinforce poor postural movements and habits that are hard to relearn.

Here are the most important elements of proper posture:

Neck. Jutting jaw or forward placement of the head is among the most common postural issues. Using machines that support the head while you do crunches or interlacing your fingers to support the

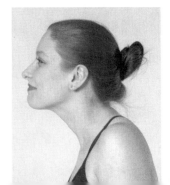

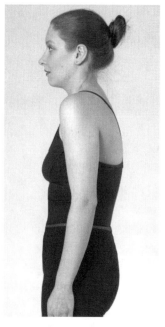

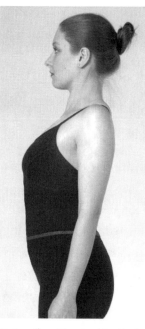

Protraction. The shoulder blades spread apart like you're hugging a tree.

Retraction. The shoulder blades are pinched together, their optimal position when you're doing upper body exercises is retracted and depressed *(see below)*.

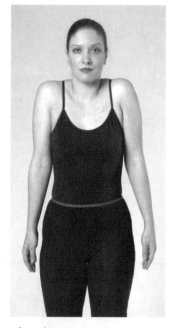

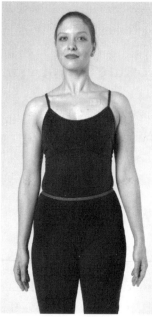

Elevation. Shoulders are up around your ears.

Depression. Shoulders are down and in a stable position.

back of your head both exacerbate the problem. If you have weak neck flexors and hold the back of your head to eliminate the stress, you're just keeping those muscles weak. At the same time, you're strengthening your abdominals. It all adds up to forward head placement.

I might be crazy, but if my forearms got sore twirling my Mom's pasta with a fork, I wouldn't stop eating the pasta; I'd make my forearms stronger! If your neck needs support when you do crunches, I suggest you do what you'd do for any other weak muscles: Strengthen them. Once you've achieved good postural form, you can follow the Neck strengthening exercises that start on page 110.

Shoulders. The shoulder girdle is one of the most complex joints of the human body. Maintaining strong, stable, flexible shoulders is necessary to your well being. But finding proper shoulder position isn't easy. In a natural, relaxed state, the shoulder blades will be in a "seated" position at the upper back. The chest will be open and wide without the points of the upper arms (shoulders) pointed forward. The tops of shoulders should also be depressed, creating a large space between them and your ears. Your shoulders can move in four primary ways: depression, elevation, protraction, and retraction.

Neutral Spine. Neutral spine, or neutral posture, is the proper alignment of the body between the postural extremes of posterior tilt and anterior tilt (right). In neutral spine, the body is able to function in its strongest, most balanced position and stress to the joints, muscles, and vertebrae is minimized. Finding and maintaining the neutral spine position helps you decrease the risk of injury and increase the efficiency of any exercises you do. The neutral spine position is different for everyone and finding it isn't always easy. Performing the Rotations (page 28) and Pelvic Tilts (page 29), which you'll find in the the PowerSculpt 10-Minute Warm-Up, will help you become aware of your pelvic movement, and that's the first step in finding your neutral spine.

Another way to find your neutral posture is to lie on your back on the floor. Bend your knees and place your feet about hip width apart and flat on the floor. You may be tempted to press your lower back into the floor, but don't. Now, place the heels of your hands on your hip bones and then place the index finger on each hand on your pubic bone. Your hands should be forming a triangle. When you're in in the neutral spine position, that triangle will be flat, parallel to the floor.

As you do the PowerSculpt Workout, keep in mind the importance of proper posture. Remember: Form is everything. Without it, not only are the exercises less effective, but they may in fact be doing harm.

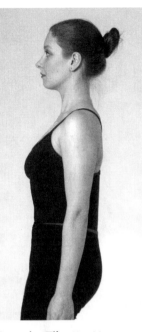

Posterior Tilt. Shoulders are rounded forward, the neck juts forward, and butt sags.

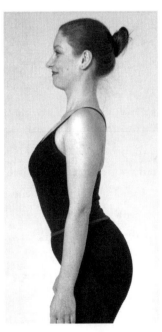

Anterior Tilt. Tight hip flexors pull your hips forward; your butt is out, and your lower back is curved inward.

PowerSculpt Tips

• When you exercise on the fitness ball, remember to **tuck your belly button into your spine.** A tight belly engages the *transverse abdominis,* the deepest of the abdominal muscles and the major stabilizer of the lower back.

• *Pain should never be part of exercise.* If you do experience pain while exercising, stop. Perhaps your posture needs to reassessed or maybe you're trying to progress too quickly.

Chapter 2

Getting Acquainted *with the* Fitness Ball

PowerSculpt is for you, no matter what your level of fitness. However, getting used to working on the fitness ball can be tricky because it's a ball and, well, balls are not stable—they tend to roll. It will take time to awaken your body's stabilizing muscles; but as your brain adapts to the stimuli it receives from your nervous system in response to training on a fitness ball, you'll learn to maintain proper posture. Once you've developed and charted your ability to stabilize yourself, you can chose the PowerSculpt Workout that's right for your fitness level. From there, you can progress to more challenging workouts. Progressing in this manner is safe and effective and will ensure that your muscles work in synergy while you perform the exercises.

Fitness Ball Basics

When you shop for a fitness ball, you'll soon discover that it's not a one-size-fits-all piece of equipment. There are several sizes available. But in the world of PowerSculpt, size matters. So here's how to choose a fitness ball that's right for you: When you sit on the ball, your thighs should be parallel to the floor and your knees bent at a 90-degree angle.

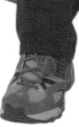

Sizing a Swiss Ball

Height	Ball Size
Up to 4'10" (145 cm)	Small 18" (45 cm)
4'10" – 5'5" (145–165 cm)	Medium 22" (55 cm)
5'5" – 6'0" (165–185 cm)	Large 26" (65 cm)
6'0" – 6'5" (185–195 cm)	X-Large 30" (75 cm)

Depending on your individual needs (sitting or exercising) you may need different sizes.

Of course, this is a rule of thumb. You can use a larger or smaller ball to change the nature of an exercise—be it a stretch or a balance or strength exercise. So once you're familiar with the workouts, experiment with different sizes—it's challenging and fun!

In addition to the ball's size, the level of inflation can change the intensity of the exercise. For PowerSculpt, I recommend keeping the ball firmly inflated, but always follow the manufacturer's directions.

Balance & Stability on the Ball

So you know which ball is right for you; now all that's left is hopping on, right? Well, not quite. Remember, this is a ball we're talking about, and when you try to simply "hop" on, it's likely to roll around a bit. That can be either annoying, unnerving, or even scary, depending on your temperament. But don't give up. All it takes is a little time and the exercises on the following pages.

Those exercises are broken out into two sets: The first three exercises will help you get onto the ball and balance with confidence. The second set of exercises allow you to gauge your stability on the ball. That's important, because knowing your level of stability lets you choose the PowerSculpt Workout that's right for you. So as you do the Stability Test moves, keep track of your progress.

13

Getting
Onto the Ball

Your first move? Sitting on the ball. When both feet are planted, you'll probably find that to be a simple task. You may find, however, that sitting comfortably with even one foot off the ground is tricky.

The Exercises

The Ball Sit, *page 15*

The Tabletop, *page 16*

The Four-Point Perch, *page 17*

The Ball Sit

If this is your introduction to the fitness ball, you will be surprised how enjoyable just sitting on the ball can be. Use it as chair at the office or at work. It will encourage good posture and engage and strengthen your core musculature.

TECHNIQUE & FORM

Place the ball next to a wall. Sit on the apex of the ball with your feet shoulder width apart. Your ears, shoulders, and hips should be in alignment. Once you feel confident, move the ball away from the wall.

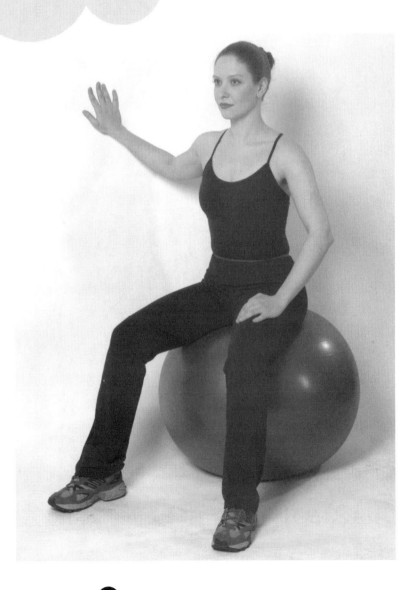

The Tabletop

The Tabletop position is an important part of a variety of chest and hip exercises. The position in itself will strengthen the hips, glutes, hamstrings, and lower back.

TECHNIQUE & FORM
Sit on the apex of the ball with your feet shoulder width apart. Slowly walk your feet forward, letting the ball roll slowly down your back to your shoulders. Stop and elevate your hips so that they're parallel to the floor. Your head and neck should be resting comfortably on the ball and your feet flat on the floor.

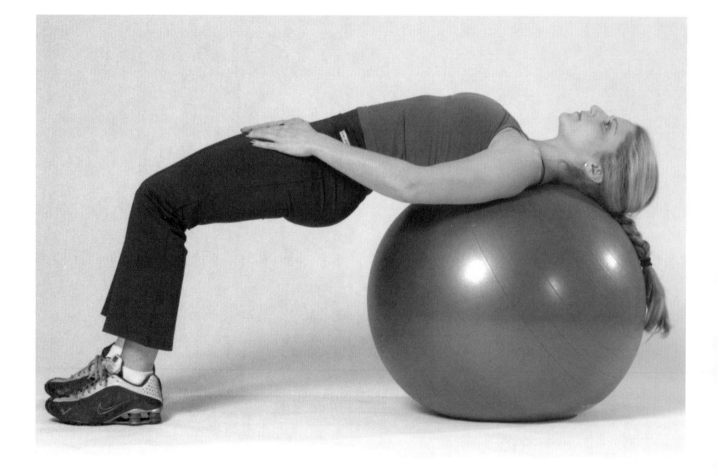

The Four-Point Perch

The Four Point Perch is the initial phase of an advanced balance position. Becoming confident and efficient in the Perch is essential before attempting advanced balance positions.

Paul's Pro Tip

If you find the *Four-Point Perch* difficult, begin with your knees on the ball and both hands on the floor. Alternate taking each hand off the floor and placing it on the ball until you're able to take both hands off the floor.

TECHNIQUE & FORM

Stand in front of the ball with your feet shoulder width apart. Gently place your knees against the ball and both hands on top of the ball. Roll forward so that your feet come off of the ground; balance in this position for as long as you feel comfortable).

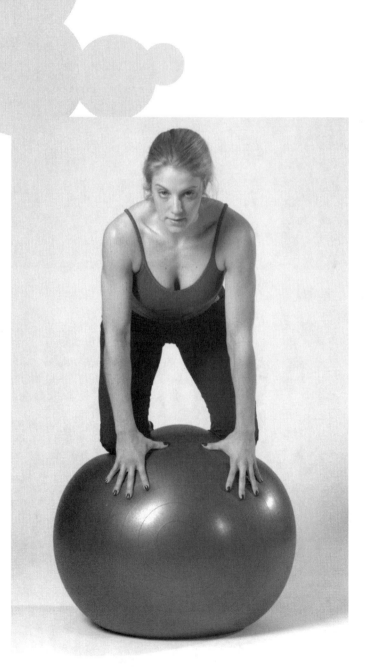

PowerSculpt
Stability
Tests

These moves will help you choose the PowerSculpt Workout level that's right for you, so be sure to keep track of how long you can hold each of these poses.

The Exercises

Shoulder Girdle Protraction, *page 19*

Shoulder Girdle Pulse, *page 20*

Back Extension, *page 21*

Reverse Back Extension, *page 22*

Hips, Buns, and Thighs Burner, *page 23*

Stability Squat, *page 24*

Single Leg Stability Squat, *page 25*

Shoulder Girdle Protraction

The **Shoulder Girdle Protraction** lets you know how strong your shoulder girdle is—and that's important information to have before you try any high-intensity upper body exercises.

TECHNIQUE & FORM

Place your knees on the ball and your hands on the floor as though you were about to do a push-up. Don't allow your hips to dip; keep your head aligned with your spine. Spread your shoulder blades as far apart as possible.

Beginner: Hold the position for 20 seconds.

Advanced: Hold the position for more than 60 seconds.

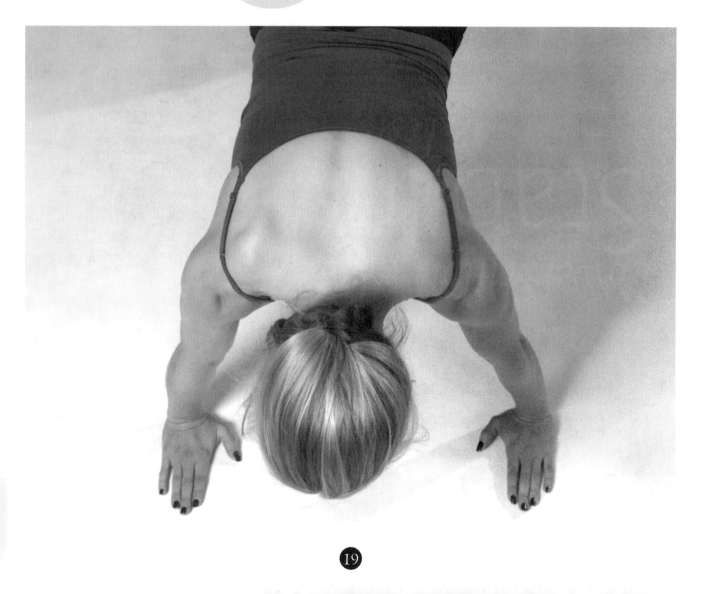

Shoulder Girdle Pulse

The **Shoulder Girdle Pulse** is a great shoulder strengthener.

TECHNIQUE & FORM

Place your knees on the ball and your hands on the floor as though you were about to do a push-up. Don't allow your hips to dip and keep your head aligned with your spine. Spread your shoulder blades as far apart as possible and then squeeze them together again.

Beginner: Do 3 sets of 10.

Advanced: Do 3 sets of 15.

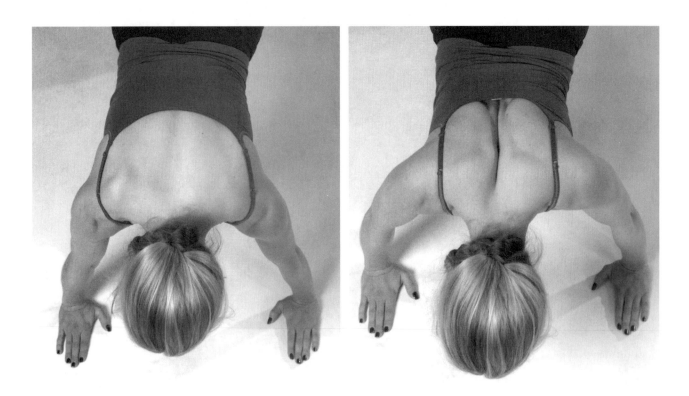

Back Extension

The back is the structural foundation of your upper body, so it's important to strengthen it—and keep it strong. The **Back Extension** will do both.

TECHNIQUE & FORM

Place the front of your hips on the ball; extend your legs behind you with your feet wide apart and your toes on the floor. Place your arms next to your sides with your palms facing the ceiling. Lift your chest off of the ball and rotate your hands toward floor. Squeeze your shoulder blades together.

Beginner: Hold the position for 30 seconds

Advanced: Hold the position for 3 minutes.

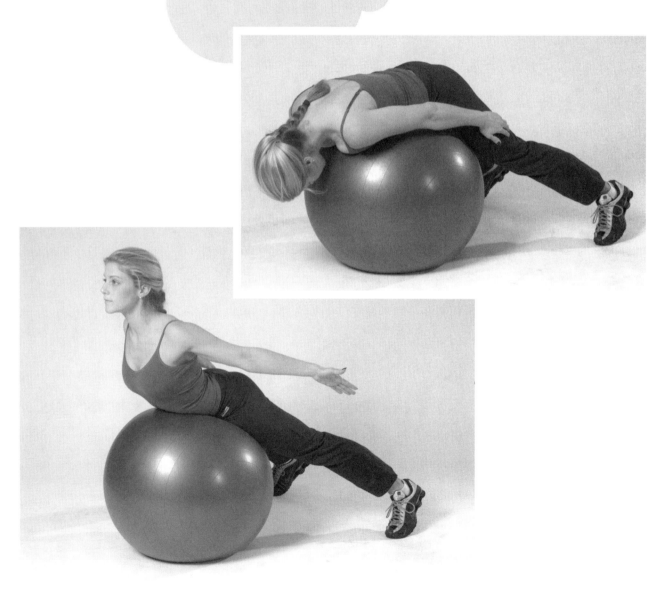

Reverse Back Extension

Test your stability on the other end with the *Reverse Back Extension.*

TECHNIQUE & FORM

Place the front of your hips on the ball and your hands and feet on the floor. Lift your legs off of the ball and hold.

Beginner: Hold the position for 30 seconds.

Advanced: Hold the position for 3 minutes.

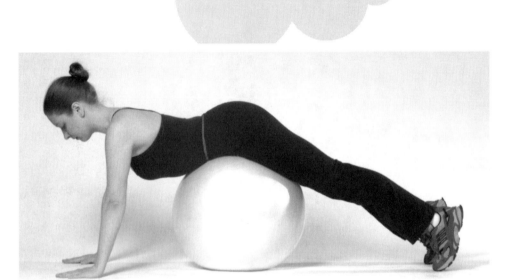

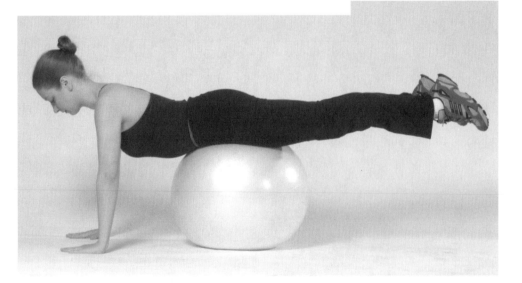

Hips, Buns, & Thighs Burner

The **Hips, Buns, & Thighs Burner** will test the strength of your "power zone," but you might do it just because it makes you look good in your jeans!

TECHNIQUE & FORM

Lie on your back on the floor; place your ankles on top of the ball. Spread your arms out to your sides with your palms down. Elevate your hips so that your ankles, hips, and shoulders are in a straight line.

Beginner: Hold the position for 30 seconds.

Advanced: Hold the position for 3 minutes.

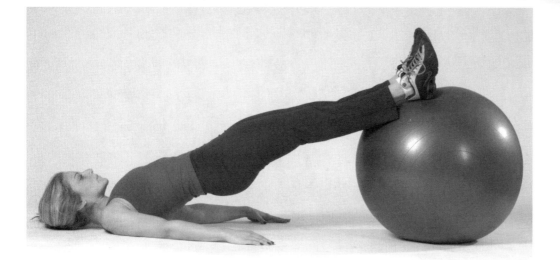

Stability Squat

The **Stability Squat** is the king of lower body exercises. In this version you won't raise and lower yourself. Instead, see how long you can hold the down position to gauge your stability.

TECHNIQUE & FORM

Stand about two feet from a wall. Place the ball between your lower back and the wall. Lower yourself until your thighs are parallel to floor. Hold yourself in the down position. **DO NOT** place your hands on top of your thighs; let them hang by your side.

Beginner: Hold position for 30 seconds.

Advanced: Hold position for 3 minutes.

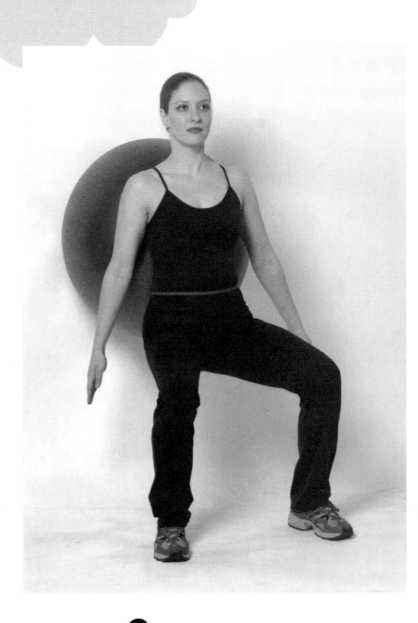

Single Leg Stability Squat

Once you've mastered the *Stability Squat* on the previous page, move on to this one, which further challenges your stability—and your quads

Paul's Pro Tip

Don't place your hands on your thighs; let them hang by your side or hold them parallel to the floor.

TECHNIQUE & FORM

Stand about two feet from a wall. Place the ball between your lower back and the wall. Lift and bend one leg at a 90-degree angle. Lower yourself until your thighs are parallel to floor and hold the position. **DO NOT** place your hands on top of your thighs; let them hang by your side.

Beginner: Hold position for 30 seconds.

Advanced: Hold position for 1 minute, 30 seconds.

Chapter 3

The PowerSculpt 10-Minute Warm-Up

Just as with any other exercise program, warming up before the PowerSculpt Workout is essential. An effective warm-up increases your heart rate and the blood flow to your muscles. That in turn increases your body temperature, which warms up your joints and enhances the elasticity of connective tissues, tendons, ligaments, and cartilage. An good warm-up increases your oxygen intake, delivering nutrients to muscles and synovial fluid to joints, which lubricates them. It will also engage the neuromuscular (balance) system, charging up reaction time and coordination.

Perform these exercises in the order they're presented for a total-body warm-up. When you're finished, you'll be ready for your PowerSculpt Workout—or any other workout, for that matter!

If you're just starting out, warming up can be a workout. Keep that in mind as you work through the exercises on the next few pages. Don't feel that you need to complete each one through the complete range of motion. Each exercise can—and should—be modified to fit your fitness level. Remember: Pain should never be part of your exercise program.

Oh, and one last thing—have fun!

The Exercises

Sitting Hip Rotations, *page 28*

Pelvic Tilts, *page 29*

Standing Rotations, *page 30*

Lunge & Rotate, *page 31*

Squat & Press, *page 32*

Jumping Jacks, *page 33*

Sit & Reach, *page 34*

Sit & Kick, *page 35*

Ax Chops, *page 36*

The Pop-Up, *page 37*

Sitting Hip Rotations

Sitting Hip Rotations are effective on several levels: They warm up and stretch your lumbar spine and engage your sense of balance. They enhance awareness of your pelvic movements, helping you discover your neutral spine.

Paul's Pro Tip

Keep your ear, shoulder, and hip in alignment and your shoulders and chest still throughout the exercise.

TECHNIQUE & FORM

Sit on the apex of the ball with your feet shoulder width apart. Place your hands on your thighs. Make small circles with your hips. Do several in each direction.

VARIATIONS

Variation I: Instead of making circles with your hips, do figure eights.

Variation II: To make this warm-up more challenging, take your hands off of your thighs and hold them parallel to the floor.

Variation III: Perform the same exercise with your feet together, then again lifting one foot off the floor.

Variation IV: Really test your balance: Do the exercise with your eyes closed!

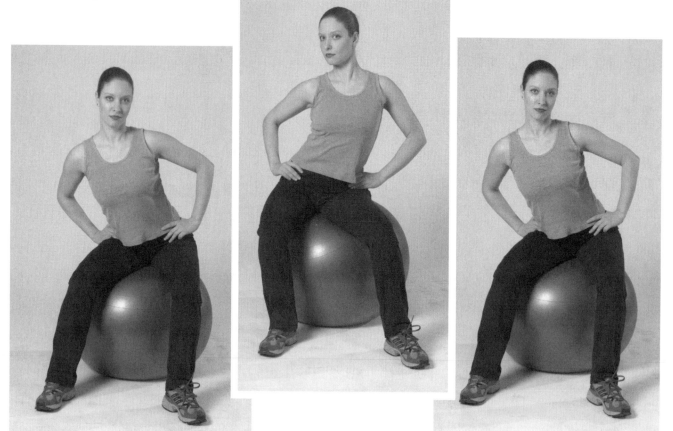

Pelvic Tilts

Pelvic Tilts are one of the simplest and most effective warm-ups and stretches for the lower back (lumbar spine).

Paul's Pro Tip

If you have trouble balancing, keep your hands on your thighs. Be sure to keep your ear, shoulder, and hip in alignment. Also, try to keep your shoulders and chest still during the exercise.

TECHNIQUE & FORM

Sit on the apex of the ball with your feet shoulder width apart. Place your hands out to your sides. Gently rock your pelvis forward and backward. (You might find you have a limited range of movement. That's okay; moving as little as 1 inch is beneficial.)

VARIATIONS

Variation I: Perform the same exercise with your feet together, then again lifting one foot off the floor.

Variation II: Do this exercise with your eyes closed to challenge your sense of balance.

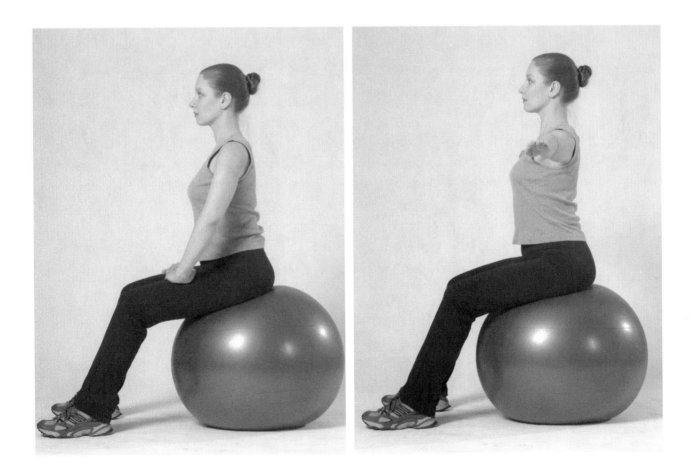

Standing Rotations

Standing Rotations are an excellent warm-up for the shoulders, waist, and hips. As you get accustomed to the movements, you'll be able to increase your range of motion.

Paul's Pro Tip
Keep your belly pulled in throughout this exercise.

TECHNIQUE & FORM
Stand with your feet shoulder width apart and your knees slightly bent. Keep your belly pulled in tight and your shoulders in their seated position. Hold the ball in your hands with your arms extended. Slowly rotate the ball in a horizontal line from right to left. Don't turn your head; keep your eyes forward. As you rotate to the right, pivot your left foot. When you rotate to the left, pivot your right foot.

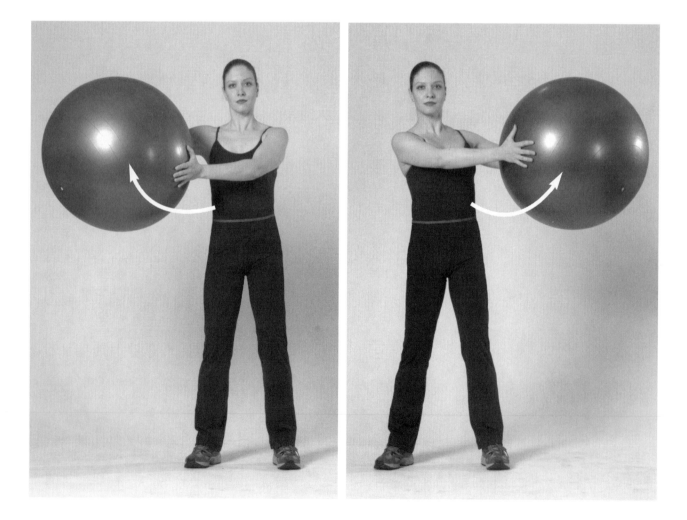

Lunge & Rotate

The Lunge & Rotate is a great full-body warm-up. It stimulates your balance and strengthens your core musculature, which stabilizes movement in your legs, hips, and shoulders.

Paul's Pro Tip

The knee of the forward leg should be directly over the ankle while you're in the lunge. Don't bang your back knee into the floor when you lunge!

TECHNIQUE & FORM

Stand with your feet together and your belly held in tightly. Hold the ball at chest height. Step forward and into a lunge with the right foot. As you do, rotate the ball over your right leg. Step back to the starting position and then lunge forward with the left leg. Alternate for the desired number of reps.

VARIATION

Hold the ball at chest height, and then swing it diagonally over the lunging leg.

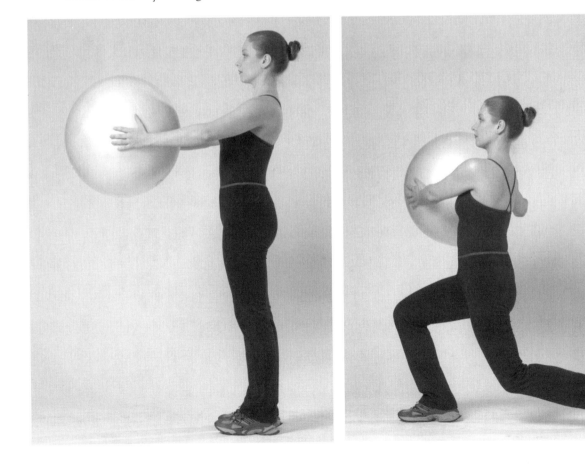

Squat & Press

The **Squat & Press** will warm you up from head to toe.

Paul's Pro Tip

Keep your back straight as you squat. To avoid straining your knees, don't let them go past your toes. If this is difficult, widen your stance and point your toes outward slightly. Those changes can help you balance and increase your range of motion.

TECHNIQUE & FORM

Stand with your chest high, your shoulders back, and your feet slightly wider than shoulder width apart. Keep your heels firmly on the ground. Hold the ball in front of you at chest level. Slowly bend your knees and lower yourself, pushing your butt back as though you're about to sit in a chair. Slowly raise yourself again, pressing the ball up over your head.

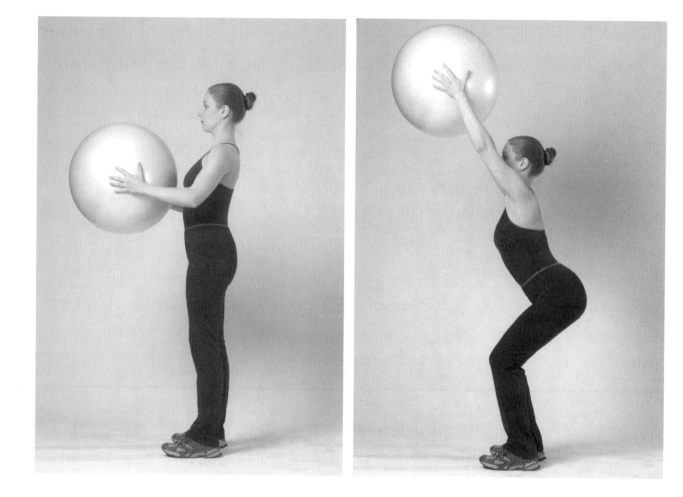

Jumping Jacks

Jumping Jacks are a fun warm-up. They'll quickly elevate your heart rate and challenge your balance and coordination.

Paul's Pro Tip
If you're having trouble balancing, keep one hand on the ball. Also, keep your back straight and avoid slouching forward.

TECHNIQUE & FORM
Sit on the apex of the ball with your feet wider than shoulder width apart. Lift your butt off the ball and drop down on it again. As you bounce, swing your arms overhead and extend your feet, raising them off the floor.

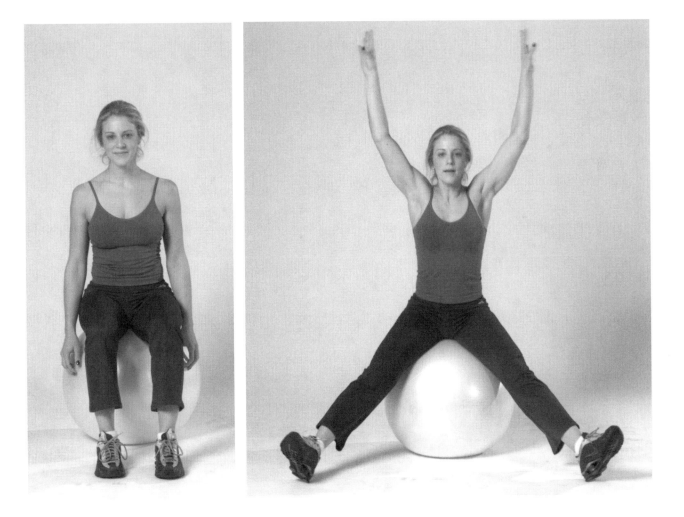

Sit & Reach

Sit & Reach engages, stretches, and warms up your waist, shoulders, and hamstrings.

Paul's Pro Tip
Stay within your range of motion; for some people this will mean simply reaching directly overhead.

TECHNIQUE & FORM
Sit on the apex of the ball with your feet wider than shoulder width apart and flat on the floor. Extend your arms out to your sides. Reach toward your left foot with your right hand. As you do so, flex your left foot. Repeat on the other side.

VARIATION
You can stretch your inner thighs and groin by placing your feet even wider apart.

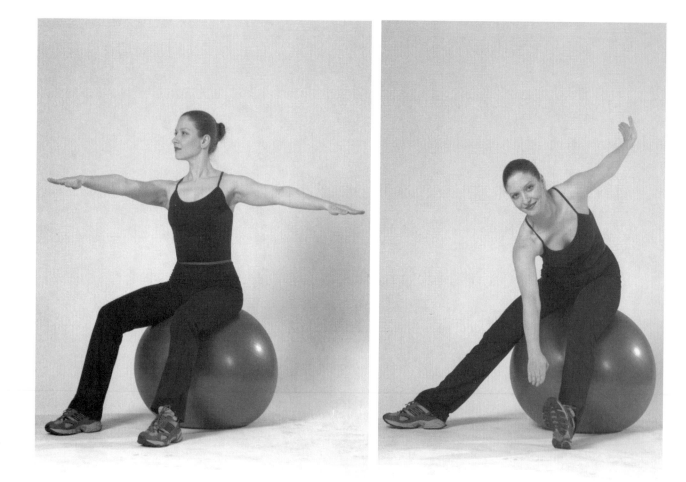

Sit & Kick

The **Sit & Kick** is a warm-up that will get your heart rate up and train the front of your thighs. But best of all you get to bounce!

Paul's Pro Tip
To prevent the ball from rolling out from under you, keep your hands on it at all times.

TECHNIQUE & FORM

Sit on the apex of the ball with your feet together and hands on the ball beside you. Lift your weight off the ball and then release, bouncing on the ball. When your weight hits the ball, it will bounce you back up. When you come back up kick out one leg. Repeat with the other leg.

VARIATION

As you kick out one leg, lift the opposite arm over your head.

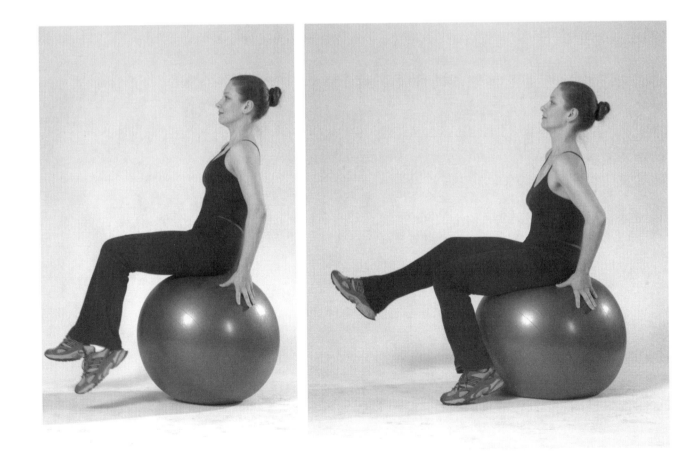

Ax Chops

Ax Chops are one of the best overall body warm-up exercises. They'll warm up and get your whole body ready for rotational movements.

Paul's Pro Tip
Keep those abs held in tightly to protect your back.

TECHNIQUE & FORM
Stand with your feet shoulder width apart and your knees slightly bent. Hold the ball over your left shoulder and then swing it diagonally to the outside of your right knee. The movement should be fast. In the finish position you'll be in a half squat with your thighs parallel to the floor. Repeat on the other side.

VARIATION
Reverse the movement, making an upward diagonal sweep.

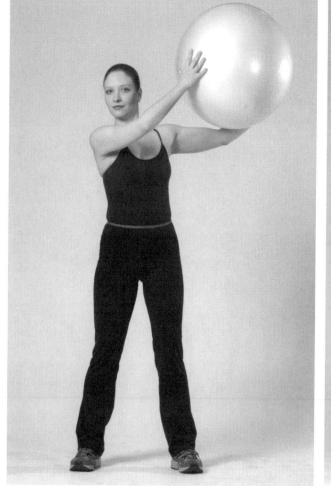
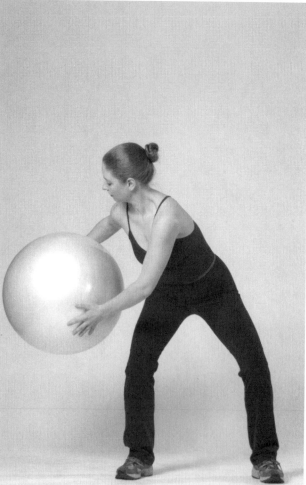

The Pop-Up

The Pop-Up is an advanced full-body warm-up and exercise. If you have any sort of back problems, you should not attempt it.

Paul's Pro Tip
You can make this warm-up a little easier by doing it more slowly and less explosively.

TECHNIQUE & FORM
Position yourself so that your toes are on the floor and you are supporting yourself on the ball with outstretched arms. Your feet should be more than shoulder width apart. Don't let your body sag—maintain your alignment. Release your body weight and bounce onto the ball. As you do come up, bring one foot alongside the ball. Bounce again and as you come up, bring the other food alongside the ball.

VARIATION
When you land, place just one hand on the ball and extend the opposite arm over your head.

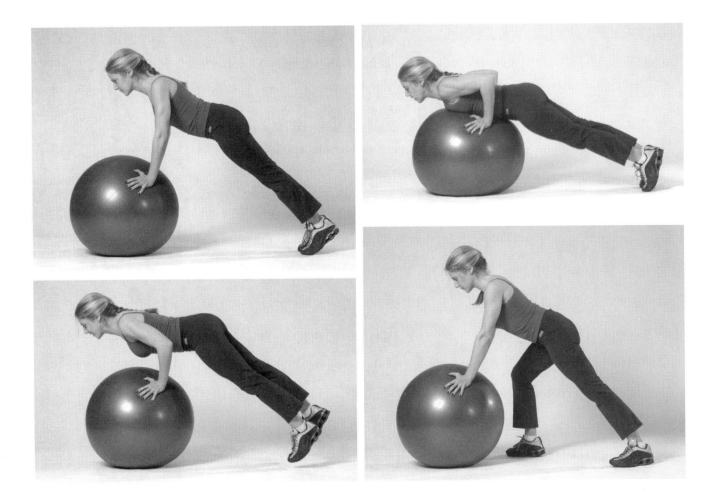

Chapter 4

The Power

After finishing the PowerSculpt Warm-Up your heart rate should be elevated; you may have even broken a slight sweat. Now you're ready for the total-body PowerSculpt moves.

The exercises are arranged by the primary muscle groups they work: chest, back, shoulders, arms, abs, legs, glutes, and even your neck. Of course, when you're working on the fitness ball, you're never working only one muscle group. When you do chest flys, for instance, you're also challenging your sense of balance and strengthening your core. Before you start, there are some bits of

Sculpt Moves

advice to keep in mind. First, always stay within your range of motion. If you can't complete the exercise as described, do what you can and gradually work up to the full movement. Remember that it's not unusual for even a fit individual to feel like a beginner the first couple of weeks working with the fitness ball. Second, stop immediately if you feel any pain. Third, remember the importance of proper form. Periodically make note of your posture and form on the ball and make adjustments if you need to.

Once you are familiar with all of the moves in this chapter, you'll be ready to move on to the *PowerSculpt* 12-Week Workouts.

PowerSculpt Chest

Pectoralis major **and** *pectoralis minor.* Training these muscles on the fitness ball will give your upper body a sleek, sculpted look and make you stronger.

The Exercises

Hands-on-Floor Push-Up, *page 41*

Leg-Lift Push-Up, *page 42*

Tippy-Toe Push-Up, *page 43*

One-Legged Toe Push-Up, *page 44*

The Clapper, *page 45*

Hands-on-Ball Push-Up, *page 46*

One-Leg-Hands-on-Ball Push-Up, *page 47*

Platform Push-Up, *page 48*

Dumbbell Flies, *page 49*

Push & Press, *page 50*

Hands-on-Floor Push-Up

When properly executed, the **Hands-on-Floor Push-Up** isn't only a chest exercise—it's also a terrific abs exercise. Doing push-ups on the ball works your core, strengthens your chest, and increases shoulder stabilization. Push-ups are among my favorite exercises because there are many variations and you can see the results so quickly.

Paul's Pro Tip

The farther away the ball is from your hips, the harder the exercise will be. It is crucial that you maintain neutral spine throughout the exercise. If your hips begin to drop, walk the ball back toward your hips to lower the intensity.

TECHNIQUE & FORM

Kneel in front of the ball, draping your hands over it. Roll out to the point of desired intensity. While in this position, (a) maintain neutral spine; (b) keep your head aligned with your spine; (c) keep your feet together on the ball; (d) keep your abs tucked in tightly (to connect the hip and shoulder). From this push-up position, lower your chest to the floor until your hands are parallel to your chest. At this point your body should be held straight. Once you can perform 10 reps without losing your form, you can progress by either adding reps or increase the intensity by rolling the ball farther away from your hips.

VARIATION

As long as you maintain your alignment and form, you can let your imagination run wild. On the following pages are just a few of the most challenging Push-Up variations.

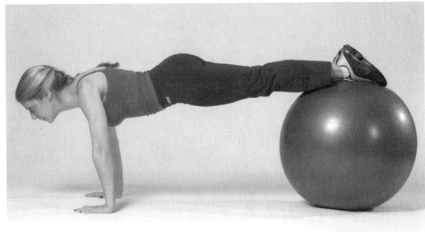

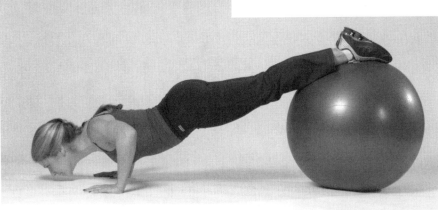

Leg-Lift Push-Up

TECHNIQUE & FORM

Kneel in front of the ball, draping your hands over it. Roll out to the point of your desired intensity. Lift one leg off the ball and lower your chest to the floor until your hands are parallel to your chest. At this point your body should be held straight.

Once you've mastered the basic Hands-on-Floor Push-Up, challenge yourself with this version.

Paul's Pro Tip

You can avoid stress on your wrists while doing all the push-ups by keeping your fingers spread wide and distributing your weight throughout your hands and fingers.

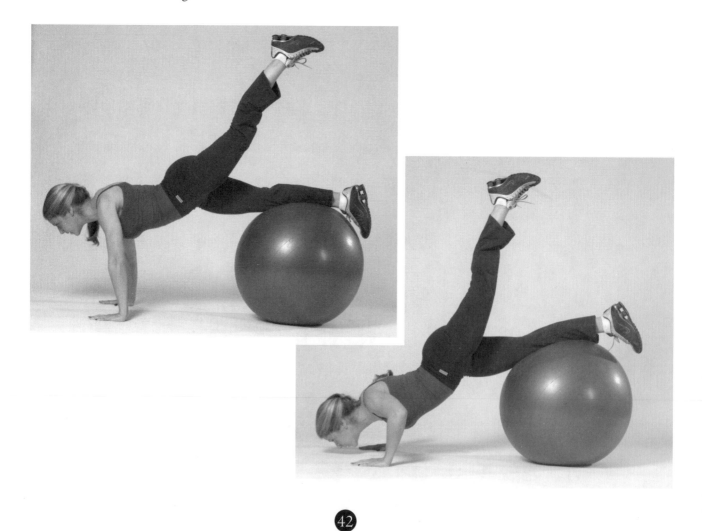

Tippy-Toe Push-Up

TECHNIQUE & FORM
Kneel in front of the ball, draping your hands over it. Roll out until your insteps are on the apex of the ball, and then lift yourself onto your toes. Lower your chest to the floor until your hands are parallel to your chest. At this point your body should be held straight.

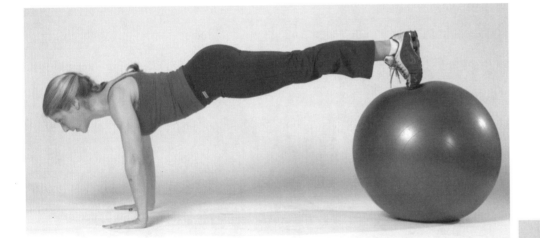

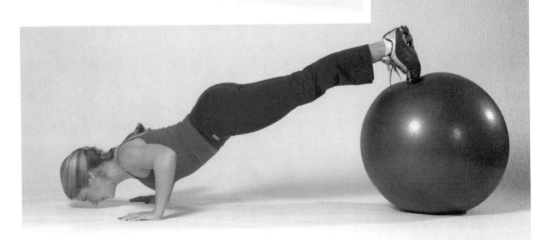

One-Legged Toe Push-Up

TECHNIQUE & FORM

Kneel in front of the ball, draping your hands over it. Roll out until your insteps are on the apex of the ball, and then lift yourself onto your toes. Lift one leg off of the ball and then lower your chest to the floor until your hands are parallel to your chest. At this point your body should be held straight.

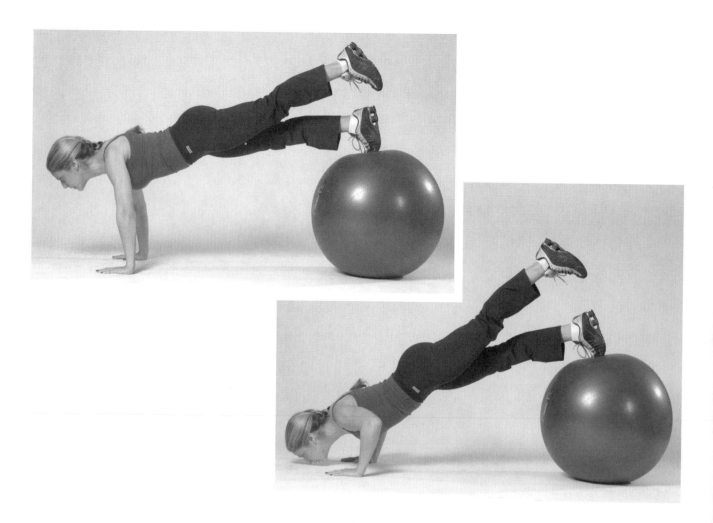

44

The Clapper

TECHNIQUE & FORM

Kneel in front of the ball, draping your hands over it. Roll out until your thighs are on the ball. Explode upward off the floor, clap your hands, and land on your hands again.

Master *The Clapper* and you'll impress all your friends. However, keep in mind that this is an advanced exercise, so don't try it until you're ready.

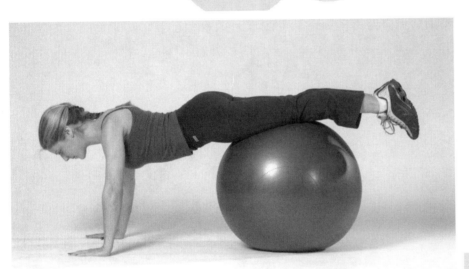

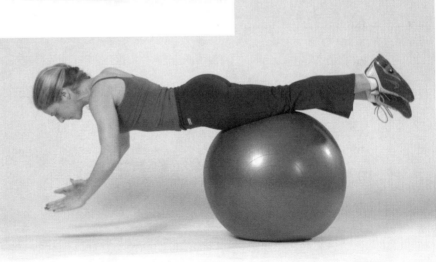

Hands-on-Ball Push-Up

As you'll discover, the **Hands-on-Ball Push-Up** is more advanced than the basic Hands-on-Floor Push-Up. It challenges your shoulder girdle and triceps.

Paul's Pro Tip
A good way to ease into this push-up is to start by setting the ball against a wall.

TECHNIQUE & FORM
Begin with your chest on the ball and your toes on the floor. Your feet should be wider than shoulder distance apart. Place your hands on the outside of the ball with your fingers pointing toward the floor. While keeping your shoulders down and in their seated position, press your chest off of the ball, and then lower yourself again.

VARIATION
Perform the push-up with your feet together.

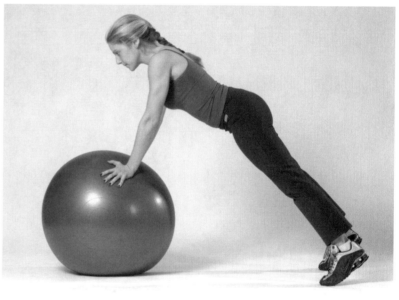

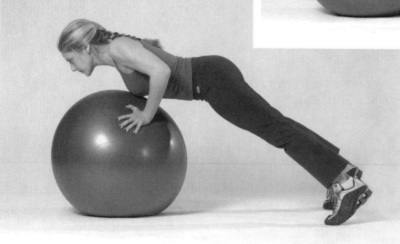

One-Leg-Hands-on-Ball Push-Up

This variation of the *Hands-on-Ball Push-Up* will really test your strength and stability.

TECHNIQUE & FORM

Begin with your chest on the ball and your toes on the floor. Your feet should be shoulder distance apart. Place your hands on the outside of the ball with your fingers pointing toward the floor. Lift one foot off the floor. While keeping your shoulders down and in their seated position, press your chest off of the ball, and then lower yourself again.

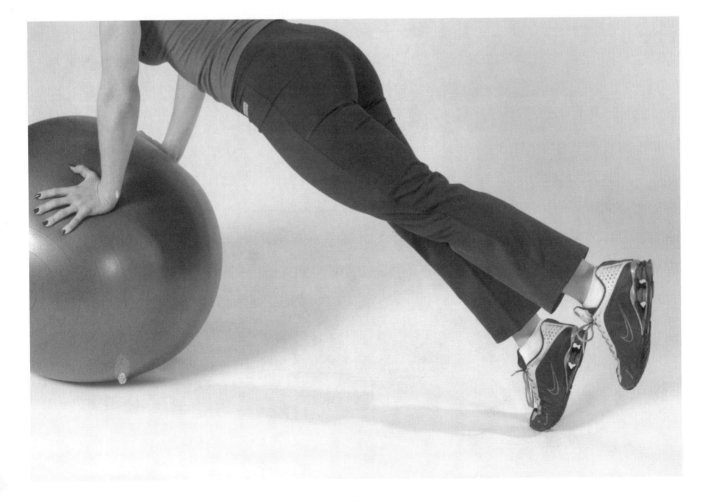

Platform Push-Up

This push-up presents a real challenge to your strength and stability. You may want to have a spotter nearby in case you lose your balance.

Paul's Pro Tip

If your hips are sagging, lower the intensity of exercise.

TECHNIQUE & FORM

Kneel on a bench and place your hands on the ball so that your fingertips point to the floor. Roll the ball out to the desired intensity. (Placing more of your leg weight on the bench lessens the intensity of the exercise.) Begin with your chest on the ball and press up to the push-up.

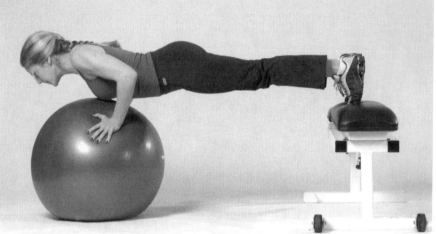

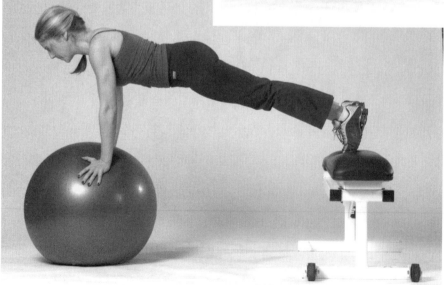

Dumbbell Flies

You can do a variety of exercises holding a weight in one or both hands. **Dumbbell Flies** sculpt and build your strength, endurance, and power, depending on the results you're looking for.

Paul's Pro Tip

When the weights meet in the middle, don't let them hit each other or even click together because at that point you're no longer working your chest muscles. If your lower back aches, drop your butt slightly.

TECHNIQUE & FORM

Start with a weight you feel comfortable lifting. Sit on the apex of the ball with your feet more than shoulder width apart. Slowly walk your feet forward, letting the ball roll slowly down your back to your shoulders. Stop and elevate your hips so that they're parallel to the floor. Your head and neck should be resting comfortably on the ball and your feet should be flat on the floor. To aid your balance, move your feet even wider apart. Extend your arms up over your chest. Keeping your elbows slightly bent, open your arms until they are parallel to floor. Bring your hands back together as though you're wrapping your arms around a tree.

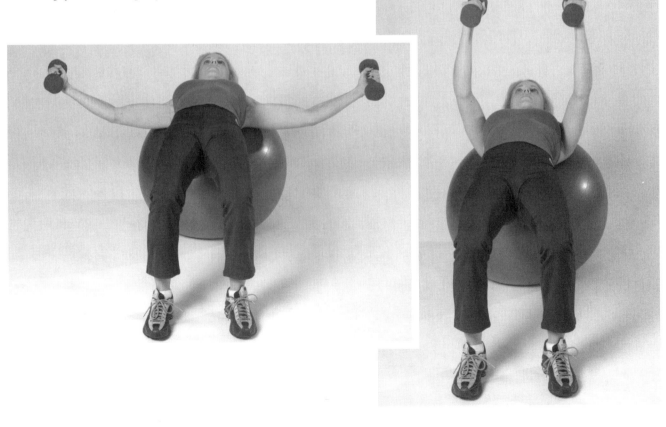

Push & Press

The **Push & Press** adds a hip extension to the usual press.

TECHNIQUE & FORM
Start with a weight you feel comfortable lifting. Sit on the apex of the ball with your feet more than shoulder width apart. Slowly walk your feet forward, letting the ball roll slowly down your back until your head, neck, shoulders, and lower back are resting on the ball. Lower the dumbbells over your chest. As you press the dumbbells up over your chest, elevate your hips so that you're in the Tabletop position. As you lower the dumbbells, lower your hips to the ball again.

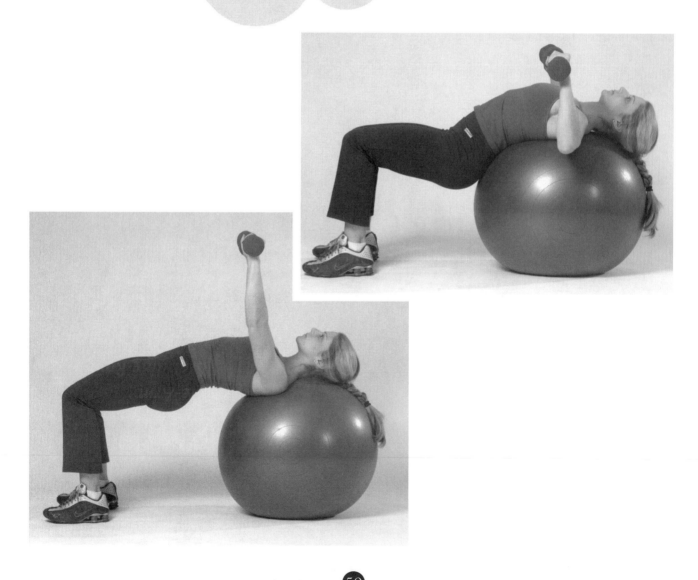

PowerSculpt Back

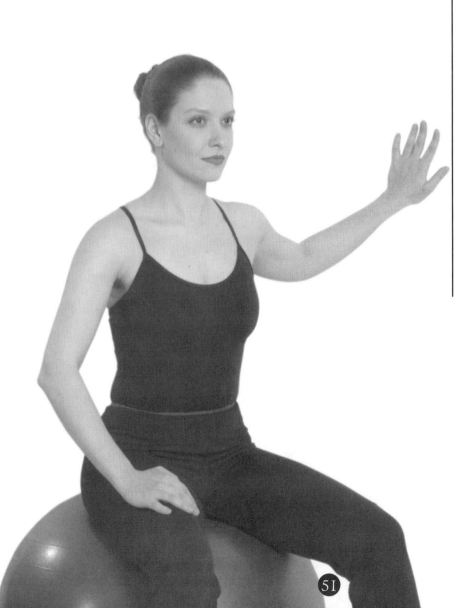

Trapezius, latissimus dorsi, rhomboids, erectors
What good is a chest that looks like a Mercedes if your back looks like a Volkswagen? Not only is a sculpted back a terrific asset in a bathing suit, but it's also the foundation of great posture.

The Exercises

Back Extension I, *page 52*

Back Extension II, *page 53*

Opposite Arm & Leg Extension, *page 54*

Reverse Back Extension, *page 55*

One-Arm Standing Row, *page 56*

Two-Point Standing Row, *page 57*

Prone Row, *page 58*

Arm Haulers, *page 59*

Pull & Press, *page 60*

Back Extension I

Instead of performing this as a stability test (as you did in the Stability Tests section), now you'll be doing **Back Extensions** to strengthen your back, holding the up position for only 3 seconds.

TECHNIQUE & FORM

Lay with your hips on the ball and your feet wide apart behind you. Keep your knees off the floor. Place your hands, palms up, by your thighs. Lift your chest off the ball, rotate your palms toward the floor, and squeeze your shoulder blades together. Hold the up most position for 3 seconds and then return to the starting position.

VARIATION

Repeat the exercise with your arms at a 45-degree angle.

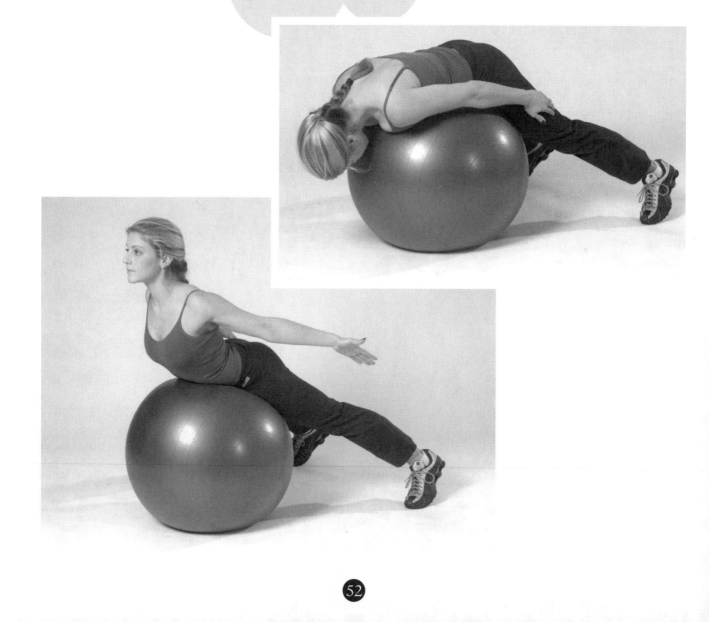

Back Extension II

The ***Back Extension II*** requires a bit more back strength and stability.

TECHNIQUE & FORM

Lay with your hips on the ball and your feet wide apart behind you. Keep your knees off the floor. Place your hands, palms up, by your thighs. Lift your chest off the ball. As you do, squeeze your shoulder blades together and extend your arms in front of you. Hold the up most position for 3 seconds and then return to the starting position.

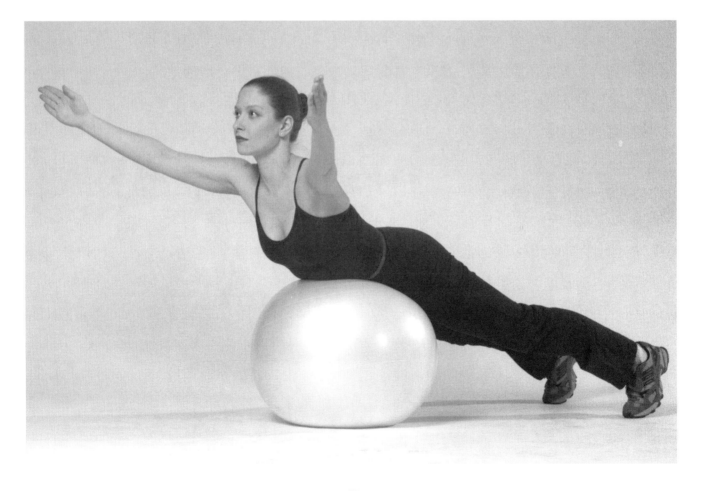

Opposite Arm & Leg Extension

TECHNIQUE & FORM

Lie with your hips on the ball and your hands and knees on the floor. Extend your left leg and your right arm until both are parallel to the floor and then switch to the other arm and leg.

This is an excellent beginner exercise for developing trunk stability.

Paul's Pro Tip

Once you feel comfortable doing this exercise, try it without the ball.

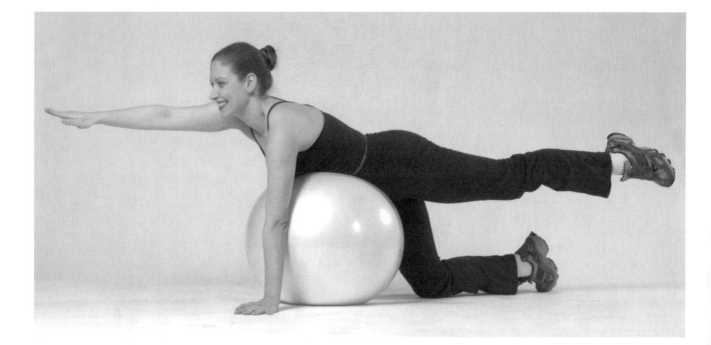

Reverse Back Extension

Here's another one you may remember from the Stability Tests section. This time you'll hold the up position for only 3 seconds.

TECHNIQUE & FORM

Place the fitness ball under the front of your hips; place your hands on the floor in front of the ball. Extend your legs behind you, with your feet hip distance apart. Keep a slight bend in your elbows. Slowly lift your legs off of the floor, keeping your knees straight, until your ankles and the back of your head are in a straight line. Hold the position for 3 seconds before returning to the starting position.

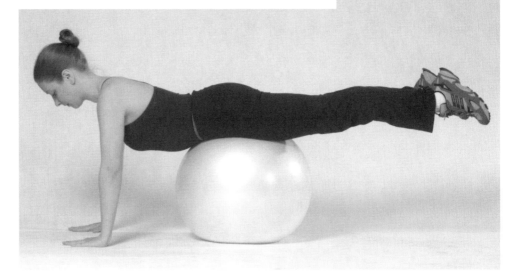

One-Arm Standing Row

The **One-Arm Standing Row** is one of the best exercises for the lats (*latissimiss dorsi*). It also doubles as an Arm exercise.

TECHNIQUE & FORM

Place the ball in front of your right foot; place your right hand on the apex of the ball. Bend slightly at the knees and at a 45-degree angle. Keep your abdominals tucked in tightly. Hold a weight in your left hand. Let the weight hang with your arm fully extended; keep your shoulder blades back, in a seated position. Pull the weight backward, allowing your elbow to lead the way, and sliding your arm along your waist. Repeat on the other side.

VARIATION

Triceps Kick Back: Place your elbow by your side (as in the finish position below) so that your upper arm is parallel to the floor. Bend and straighten your elbow to work the triceps muscles.

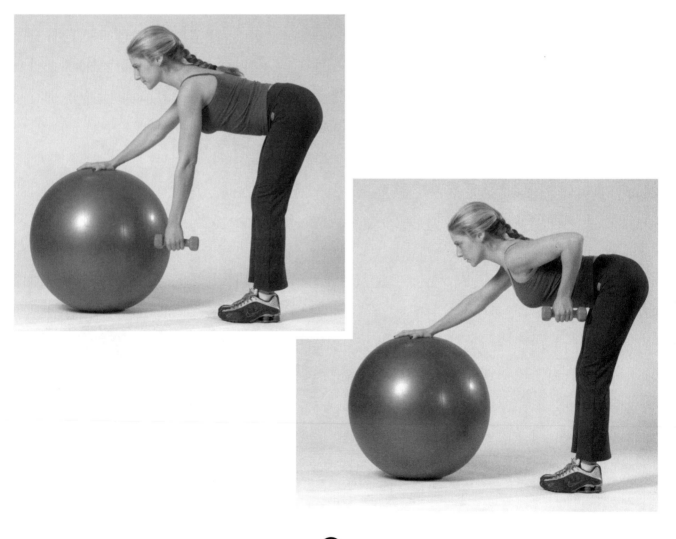

Two-Point Standing Row

The **Two-Point Standing Row** challenges your stability *and* sculpts your lats.

TECHNIQUE & FORM

Place the ball in front of your right foot; place your right hand on the apex of the ball. Hold a weight in your left hand. Let the weight hang with your arm fully extended; keep your shoulder blades back, in a seated position. Elevate and extend your right leg behind you. Slightly bend your left leg and pull the weight backward, allowing your elbow to lead the way, and sliding your arm along your waist. Repeat on the other side.

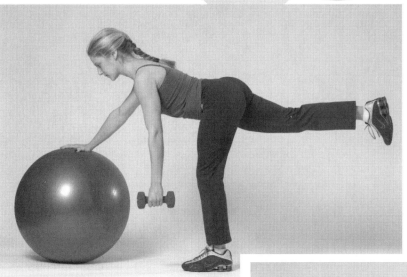

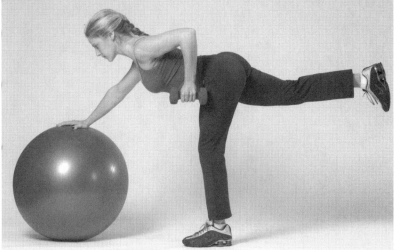

Prone Row

The **Prone Row** targets the upper back and shoulders. Making those muscles strong will correct unattractive forward slouching shoulders and give you a fine straight-back look.

Paul's Pro Tip

When you lie on the ball, make sure you're in a position that doesn't impede your breathing. Avoid the tendency to elevate your shoulders while you do this exercise.

TECHNIQUE & FORM

Lie with your chest on the ball; extend your legs behind you with your feet about shoulder width apart. Hold a dumbbell in each hand. Keeping your chest elevated, pull the weights back with your arms at a 90-degree angle. Keep your shoulders in the seated position and squeeze your shoulder blades together.

VARIATION

Perform the exercise one arm at a time.

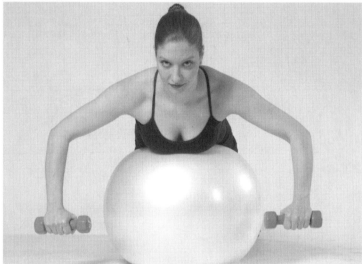

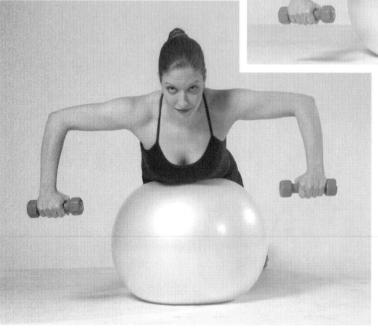

Arm Haulers

This one works your shoulders
and upper back, too.

TECHNIQUE & FORM

Start with a weight you feel comfortable lifting. Lie with your chest on the ball, your toes on the floor, and the weights at your sides. Keep your head aligned with your spine to avoid stressing your neck. Move the weights from your hips to out in front of you, in a circular motion.

VARIATION

These are challenging if you do them with no weight but lots of reps.

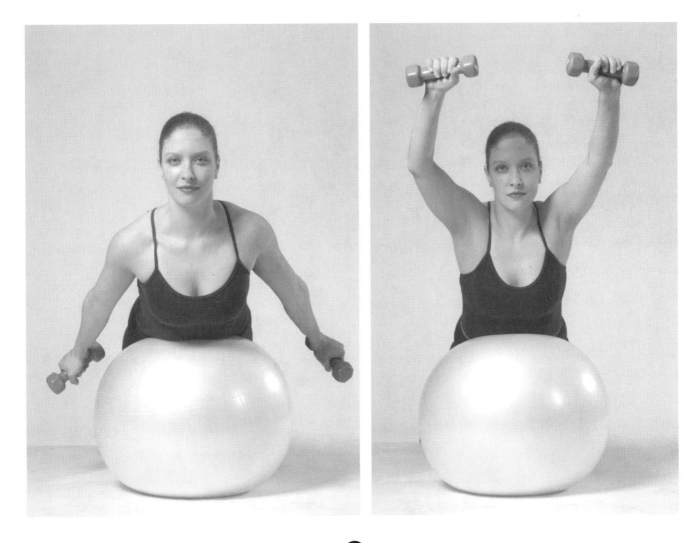

Pull & Press

The **Pull & Press** strengthens the hips, glutes, abs, shoulders, and chest.

Paul's Pro Tip

The most common mistake people make when they do these kinds of exercises is hyper-extending their hips in the topmost position. That can cause lower pack pain; so always exercise within a pain-free range of motion.

TECHNIQUE & FORM

Start with a dumbbell that you feel comfortable lifting. Sit on the apex of the ball with your feet shoulder width apart. Slowly walk your feet forward, letting the ball roll down your back until it reaches your shoulders. Drop your butt to floor and hold the weights over your head.

As you lift your butt off the floor, lift the weights to your hips. Keep your abs engaged at all times. As you lower your butt, lower the weights again over your head.

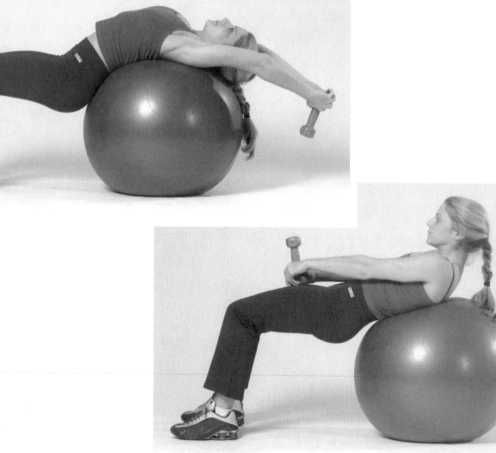

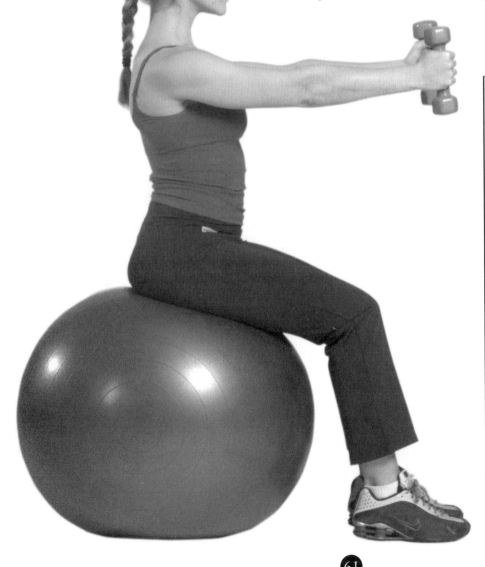

PowerSculpt
Shoulders

Anterior, medial, and *posterior* deltoids

Sculpted, shapely shoulders. Sounds good, doesn't it? Well to get the sexy shoulders you want, you need to target your shoulder muscles (deltoids) on three different planes: the side (lateral), the rear (posterior) and the front (anterior) of the shoulder. And the exercises on the following pages do just that.

As you perform each of these exercises, keep several points in mind: (1) Always maintain proper shoulder position thought the full range of motion; (2) begin with light weights; and (3) never lift the weight above shoulder height if you have shoulder problems.

The Exercises

Fly & Hug, page 62

Seated Lateral Raise, page 63

Waist-on-Ball Lateral Raise, page 64

Seated Overhead Press, page 65

Seated Posterior Extension, page 66

Waist-on-Ball Posterior Extension, page 67

Anterior Raise, page 68

Two-Point Anterior Raise, page 69

Fly & Hug

The ***Fly & Hug*** takes the usual chest fly to a new level, strengthening the chest and rear shoulder.

Paul's Pro Tip
Do this exercise with a light weight, because your chest muscles will be much stronger than the rear shoulder.

TECHNIQUE & FORM

Sit on the apex of the ball with your feet shoulder width apart. Slowly walk your feet forward, letting the ball roll down your back until it reaches your shoulders. Stop and elevate your hips so that they're parallel to the floor. Your head and neck should be comfortably resting on the ball. Do a chest fly, but instead of stopping when your hands meet in the middle, continue the movement until the weights touch the opposite shoulder.

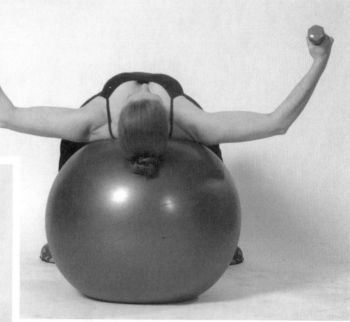

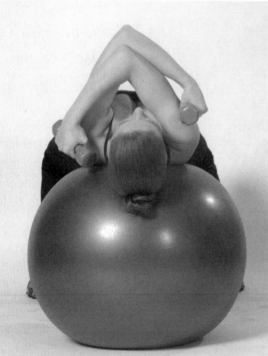

Seated Lateral Raise

TECHNIQUE & FORM
Sit on the apex of the ball. Maintain proper posture and keep your feet flat on the floor. Hold the dumbbells (palms down) by your sides, letting them rest on the side of the ball. Keeping your elbows bent slightly, slowly lift the dumbbells out to your sides and to shoulder height. Lower them again, but don't let them rest on the ball again.

Avoid this exercise if you have shoulder problems.

Paul's Pro Tip
If you prefer, lift or press the weights over your head instead of raising them laterally.

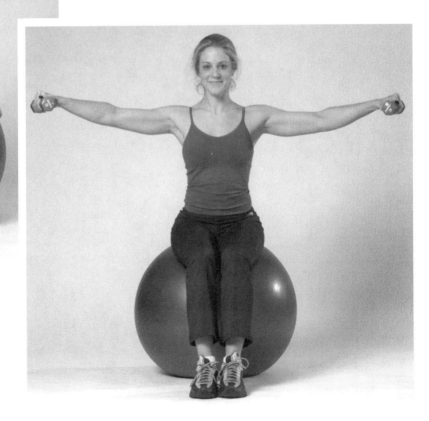

Waist-on-Ball Lateral Raise

You may need to use a smaller ball to do this exercise.

TECHNIQUE & FORM

Lie with your hips and waist on the ball. The hand of the bottom arm should be flat on the floor. Hold the dumbbells (palms down) by your side. Keeping your elbows bent slightly, slowly lift the dumbbells to shoulder height and then lower them again, but don't let them rest on your side again.

Seated Overhead Press

The **Seated Overhead Press** works your arms and your shoulders, all while challenging your stability on the ball.

TECHNIQUE & FORM
Sit on the apex of the ball with your chest high and shoulders back. Holding the weights with both hands, press them over your head and then lower them again.

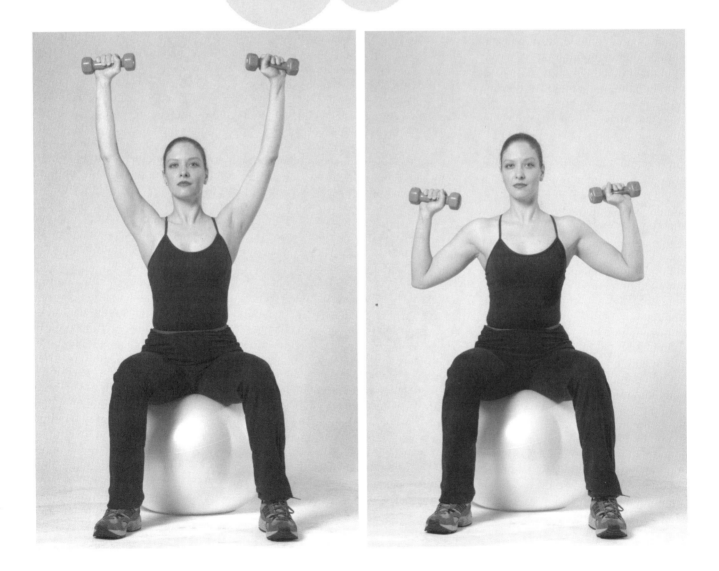

Seated Posterior Extension

The posterior deltoid is typically the weakest of the three shoulder muscles because it is difficult to isolate. To properly target these rear shoulder muscles lighten up the weight, so you use correct form.

TECHNIQUE & FORM

Sit on the apex of the ball. Maintain proper posture and keep your feet flat on the floor. Hold the dumbbells (palms facing inward) by your side. Bend at the waist so that your chest comes close to your knees and the weights are by your ankles. Lift the weights until they're parallel to the floor. Slowly lower them back to the starting position and repeat.

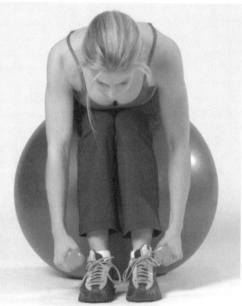

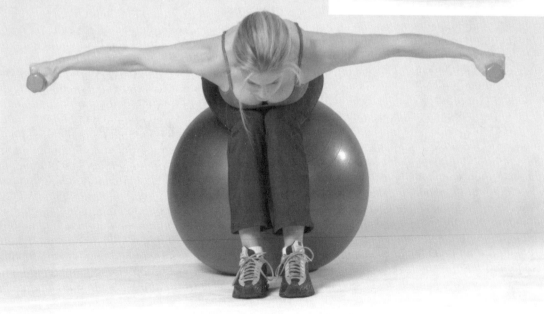

Waist-on-Ball Posterior Extension

As with the other waist-on-ball exercises, you may have to switch to a smaller ball to maintain correct form.

TECHNIQUE & FORM

Lie with your hips and waist on the ball. The hand of the bottom arm should be flat on the floor. Extend the top arm straight out in front of you, holding the weight palm-down. Keeping your elbows bent slightly, slowly lift the dumbbells over your head and then slowly lower it again.

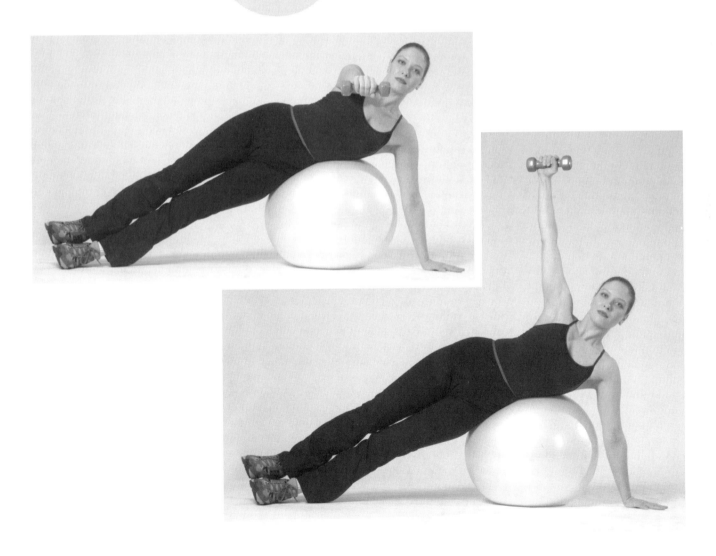

Anterior Raise

To properly execute the **Anterior Raise** focus on keeping the shoulder blades in a seated position and avoid swinging the weight.

Paul's Pro Tip

With all the shoulder exercises maintaining proper shoulder position through the full range of motion is essential—as is beginning with light weights.

TECHNIQUE & FORM

Sit on the apex of the ball. Maintain proper posture and keep your feet flat on the floor. Hold the dumbbells (palms facing inward) by your side, letting them rest on the side of the ball. Lift the weights in front of you to shoulder height. Hold for a second before lowering the weights back to the staring position; repeat.

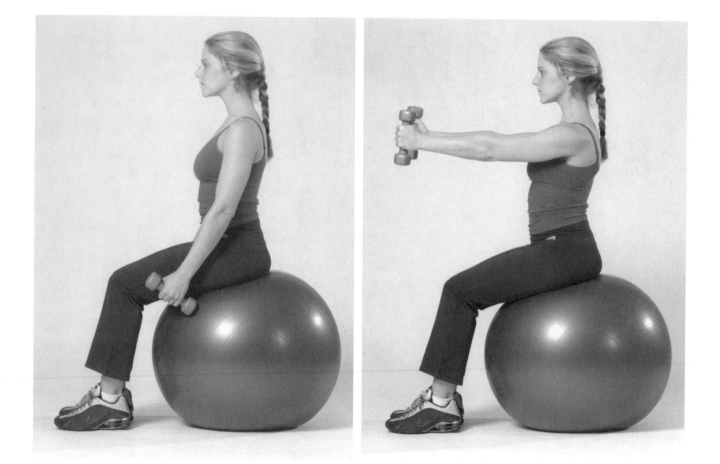

Two-Point Anterior Raise

To perform the **Two-Point Anterior Raise** without losing your balance, it's important to do it slowly.

TECHNIQUE & FORM

Kneel on the apex of the ball. Hold the dumbbells (palms facing inward). Lift the weights in front of you to shoulder height. Hold for a second before lowering the weights back to the starting position; repeat.

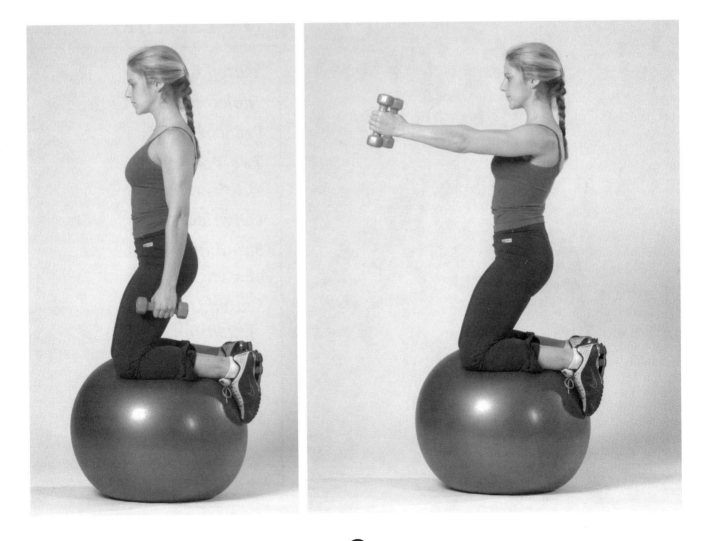

PowerSculpt Arms

Biceps Brachii and **Triceps Brachii**

Do you have a little jiggle under your arms? Do your arms get tired holding a bag of groceries for more than a couple of minutes? Are you dreading swimsuit or tank top season? Then the PowerSculpt moves on the next several pages are the answer!

The Exercises

Seated Biceps Curls, *page 71*

Tabletop Biceps Curls, *page 72*

Preacher Curls, *page 73*

Two-Point Biceps Curls, *page 74*

Long Head Press, *page 75*

Standing Triceps Extensions, *page 76*

Seated Overhead Extension, *page 77*

Tabletop Triceps Extensions, *page 78*

Seated Dip, *page 79*

Seated Biceps Curls

Another classic exercise paired with the fitness ball. As your strength and balance improve you'll be able to move to heavier weights—and the Two-Point Biceps Curls.

TECHNIQUE & FORM

Start with a weight you feel comfortable lifting. Sit on apex of the ball with your feet flat on the floor. Keep your chest high and your shoulders back. Let the weights hang by your sides, resting on the ball. Raise the weights with your palms facing your shoulders. Lower them, but don't let them rest on the ball again.

VARIATION

Do the biceps curl with only one foot on the floor. This intensifies the exercise by incorporating your leg and trunk muscles.

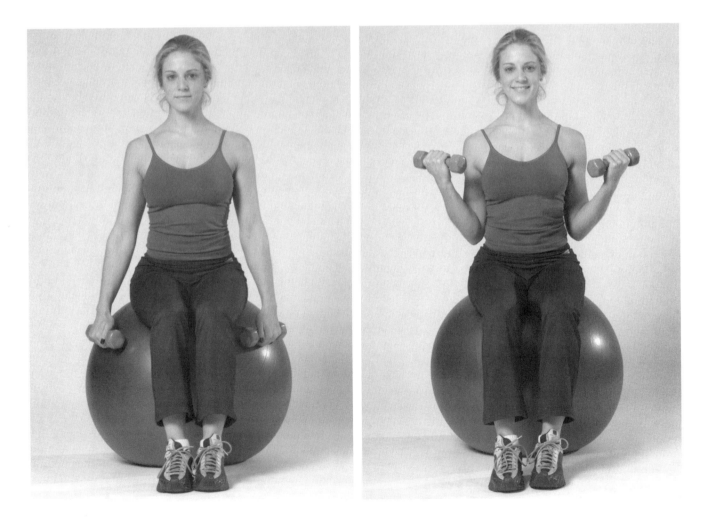

Tabletop Biceps Curls

Don't be surprised if you
need to use a lighter weight
than you used for the
Seated Biceps Curls.

TECHNIQUE & FORM

Sit on apex of the ball, and then roll down to the Tabletop position, allowing your lower back to remain on and be supported by
the ball. Your elbows and the back of your upper arms should rest
comfortably on the ball. Let the weights hang freely with your
arms fully extended; you will most likely feel a stretch of the
biceps muscle. Lift the weight toward the top of your shoulder in a
full range of motion, and then return to bottom position.

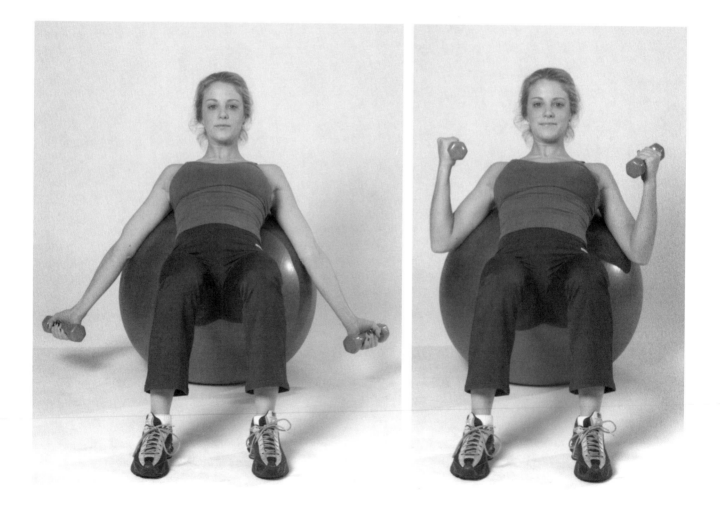

Preacher Curls

I'm not sure how these got their name, but *Preacher Curls* are terrific for isolating and sculpting your biceps.

TECHNIQUE & FORM

Start with a weight you feel comfortable lifting. Kneel behind the ball, resting your triceps on its apex. Maintain your stability as you perform curls with one or both arms.

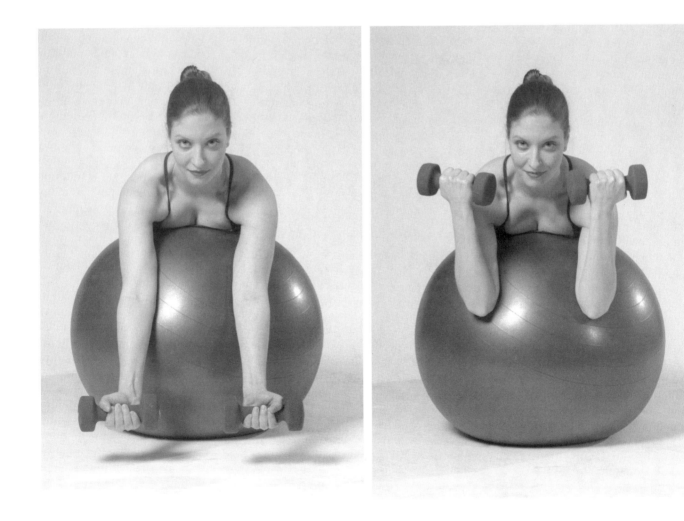

Two-Point Biceps Curls

This is an advanced exercise and one that you shouldn't attempt unless you're completely confident in your ability to maintain a two point stance on the ball.

TECHNIQUE & FORM

Approach the ball with the weights in your hands. Place your knees and hands on the ball and roll to a four-point stance (aka The Perch, page 17). Lift yourself to a two-point stance. Maintain stable hips as you do biceps curls. Try curls working one arm at a time and then both arms at once.

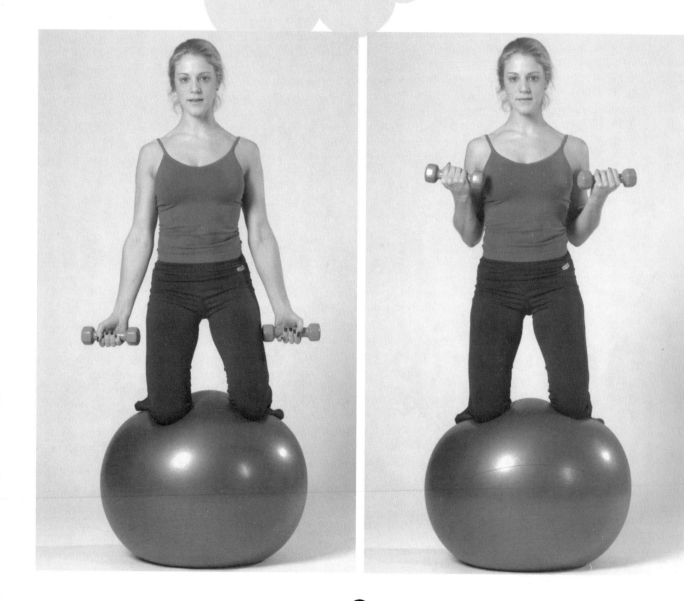

Long Head Press

TECHNIQUE & FORM

Start with a weight you feel comfortable lifting. Sit on the apex of the ball with your feet more than shoulder width apart. Slowly walk your feet forward, letting the ball roll slowly down your back to your shoulders. Stop and elevate your hips so that they're parallel to the floor. Your head and neck should be resting comfortably on the ball and your feet should be flat on the floor. Keeping your shoulder blades pressed back, press the weights up over your chest. Keep the weights in line with your elbows.

The **Long Head Press** recruits heavily from your triceps.

Paul's Pro Tip

If you're having trouble balancing, move your feet wider apart. Keep your shoulder blades pressed together tightly to better target your chest muscles.

Standing Triceps Extension

This exercise is an old favorite done with the fitness ball. The benefit? In addition to sculpting your triceps, you'll be improving your balance and stability.

TECHNIQUE & FORM

Start with a weight you feel comfortable lifting. Stand with your legs slightly bent, one hand on the ball, and the weight in your free hand. Lift your arm behind you until your upper arm is parallel to the floor. Straighten and bend your elbow.

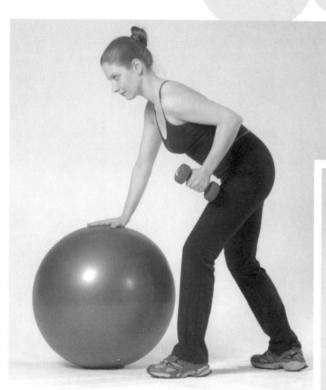

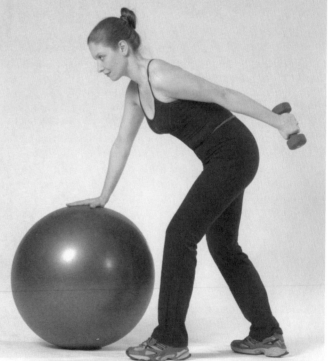

Seated Overhead Extension

The triceps muscle can be tricky to isolate but this classic exercise will do the trick. Make sure that you keep your elbows close to your head at all times.

TECHNIQUE & FORM

Start with a weight you feel comfortable lifting. Sit on the apex of the ball. Hold the dumbbell with both hands and place it over your head. Keeping the elbows parallel with each other, lower the weight behind your head with your forearms until your elbows are bent at a 90-degree angle. Press up with your forearms using the triceps muscle. Keep the elbows slightly bent in the topmost position.

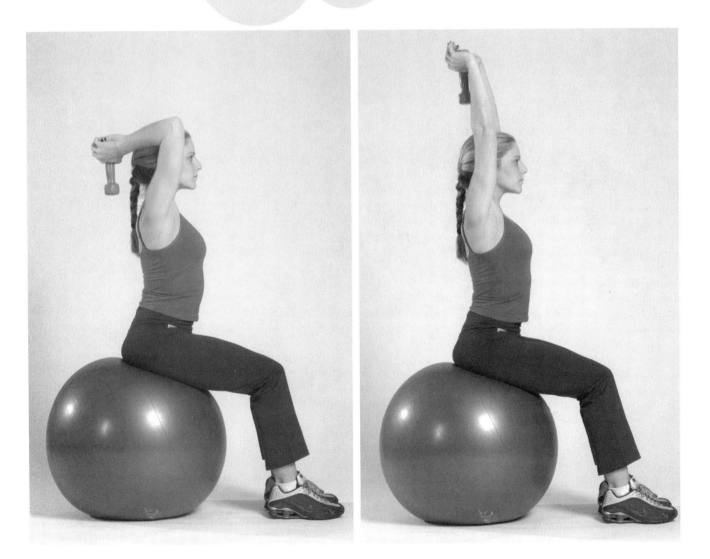

Tabletop Triceps Extensions

One of the best things about owning a fitness ball is that it stands in for other pieces of gym equipment. For instance, you'd normally need a weight bench at home to do this exercise.

TECHNIQUE & FORM

Start with a weight you feel comfortable lifting. Sit on the apex of the ball and roll down to the Tabletop position. Once there, extend your arms over your chest. Bend your arm at the elbow, lowering the weights so that they're parallel to the floor.

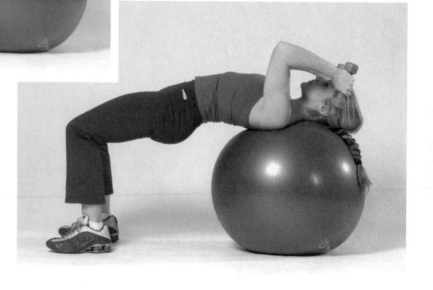

Seated Dip

Another classic triceps exercise updated with the fitness ball!

Paul's Pro Tip

Once you've mastered this one, try it while lifting one leg off the ball.

TECHNIQUE & FORM

Sit on a bench and place your ankles on the ball. Keep your fingers pointed forward, toward the ball. Lift your hips off of the bench and lower your body until your elbows are bent at a 90-degree angle. Raise yourself again.

VARIATION

Sit on the ball and place your hands next to your butt. Lift yourself off the ball and drop your hips toward the floor.

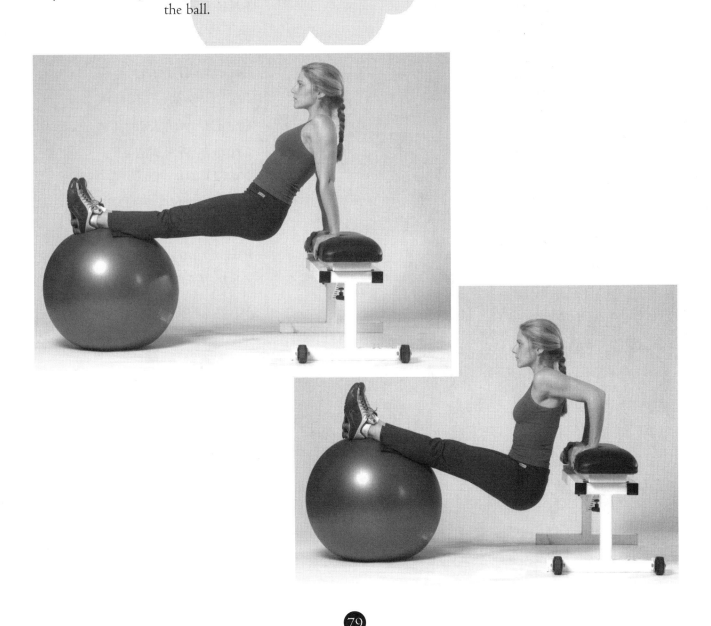

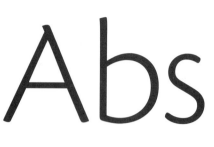

Abs

Rectus abdominis, external obliques, and internal obliques

No other muscles are as sexy as the abs. That's why most of us are obsessed with having a lean, tight, flat, and curvy waistline. To properly work your abs, you need to train them using a variety of movements: flexion, extension, and rotation. Training your abs on a fitness ball engages even more muscle fiber—more muscle fibers engaged means more muscles sculpted.

Sure, we all want to look good, but being sexy isn't only about looking good; it's about being strong and self-confident, too. Putting in an eight-hour day, picking up kids, and doing yard work all require strong abs. If you want to be sexy and strong, then don't ignore your abs.

The Exercises

Crunch, *page 81*

Reverse Crunch, *page 82*

Crunch with Rotation, *page 83*

Crunch with Knee Curl, *page 84*

Crunch with Knee Side Curl, *page 85*

Body Crunch, *page 86*

The Pike, *page 87*

Pike Crunch, *page 88*

Ab Roll, *page 89*

Scissor Rotations, *page 90*

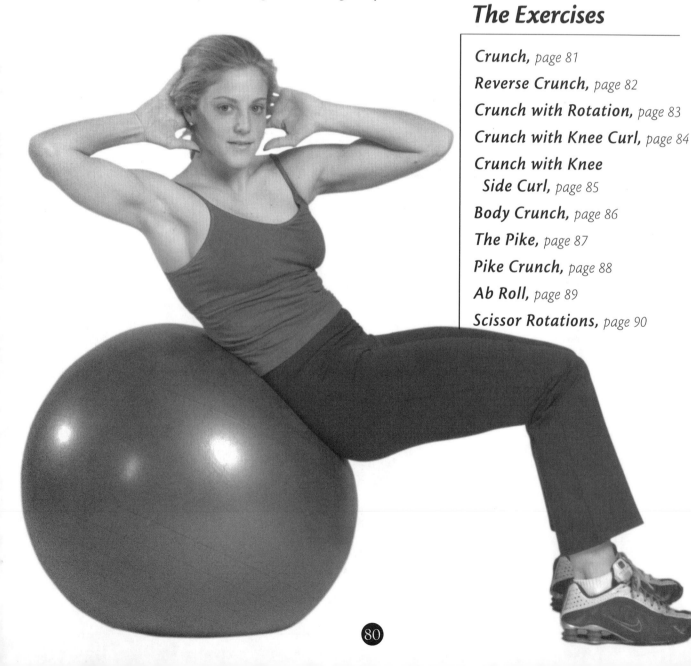

Crunch

Doing crunches on the fitness ball increases the range of motion through which your abs must work. That makes the fitness ball *Crunch* a much more effective exercise.

TECHNIQUE & FORM

Sit on the apex of the ball with your feet shoulder width apart. Walk your feet forward until your lower back is firmly supported. Place your fingers by your temples; keep your elbows wide. Lower your upper back and shoulders onto the ball. Lift your upper back and shoulders off the ball to a roughly 45-degree angle. Keep your hips anchored so that you move over the ball, and the ball does not roll under you.

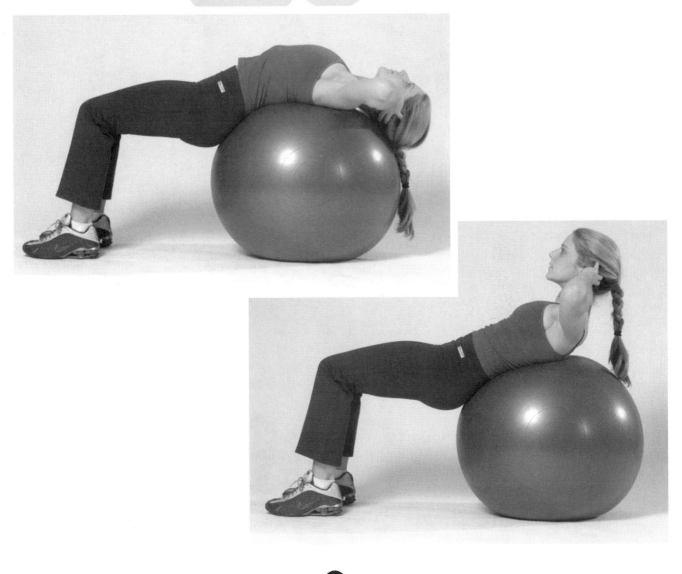

Reverse Crunch

The **Reverse Crunch** targets the hard-to-engage lower abdominals.

Paul's Pro Tip
If you feel discomfort in your lower back, don't lower the ball all the way to the floor.

TECHNIQUE & FORM
Lie on your back on the floor with your knees bent and legs on the ball. The ball should be wedged between your butt and calves. Lift the ball off the floor with your heels and draw your knees to your chest and then slowly return them to the floor.

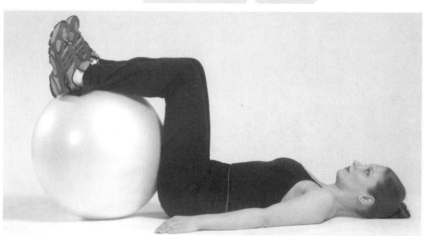

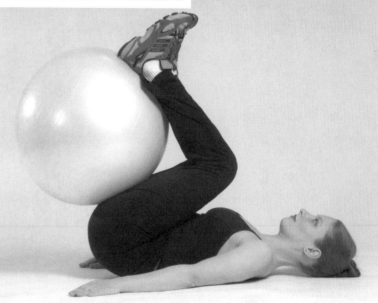

Crunch with Rotation

The ***Crunch with Rotation*** adds a twist that engages your obliques.

TECHNIQUE & FORM

Sit on the apex of the ball with your feet shoulder width apart. Walk your feet forward until your lower back is firmly supported. Place your fingers by your temples; keep your elbows wide. Lower your upper back and shoulders onto ball. Lift your upper back and shoulders off the ball to a roughly 45-degree angle. As you do, turn your torso to the left, and then lower yourself. Repeat, switching sides.

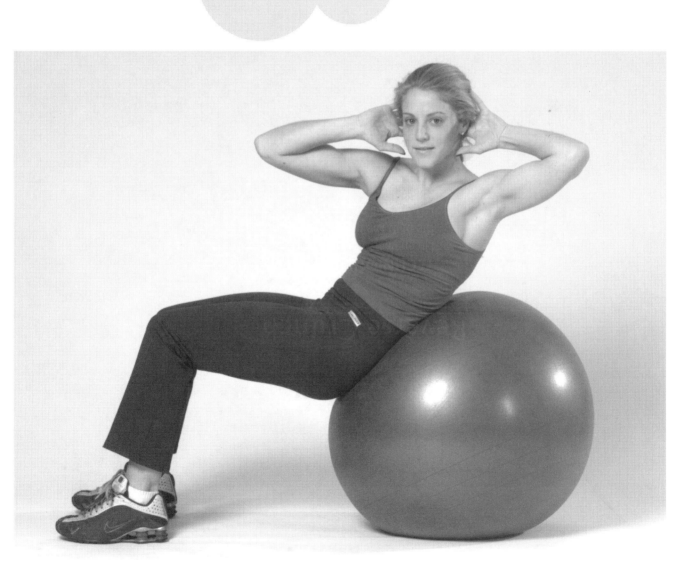

Crunch with Knee Curl

TECHNIQUE & FORM

Lay on your hips on the ball. Walk your hands out until your insteps are on the ball's apex. Pull the ball into your chest and then roll it out again.

The **Crunch with Knee Curl** strengthens the lower abdominal region and your shoulders.

Paul's Pro Tip

It's important to keep your hips elevated while you draw your knees into your chest.

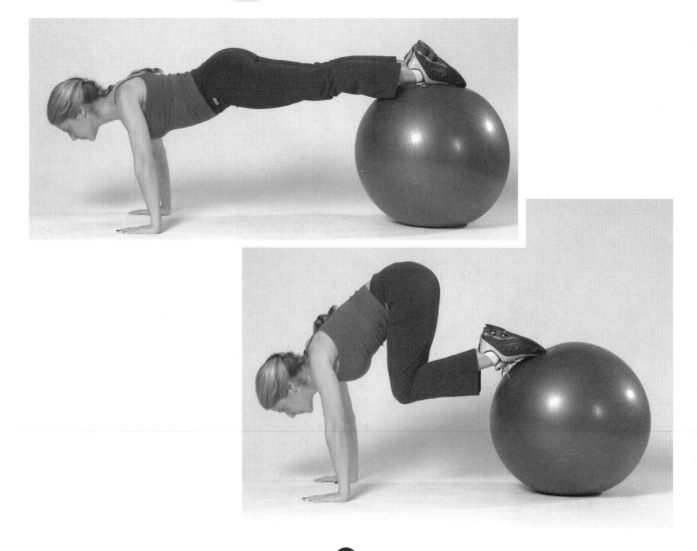

Crunch with Knee Side Curl

This crunch requires strong shoulder stabilization and waist rotation.

TECHNIQUE & FORM

Lay on your hips on the ball. Walk your hands out until your insteps are on the ball's apex. Pull the ball into toward one shoulder, then roll it out again. Repeat, moving the ball toward the opposite shoulder.

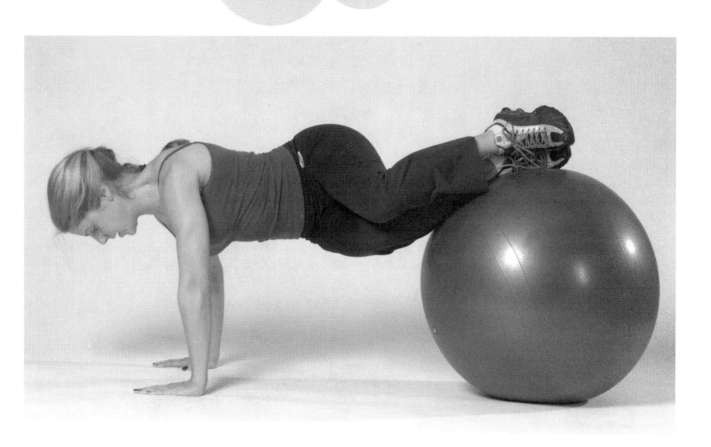

Body Crunch

This crunch works your inner thighs and your abs.

Paul's Pro Tip
Focus on tucking your abs into your spine while you're doing this (or any) ab exercise.

TECHNIQUE & FORM
Lie on the floor with your knees bent and the ball between your calves. Place your fingertips on your temples. Lift your shoulder blades off the floor and simultaneously squeeze the ball with your calves. Slowly lower yourself again.

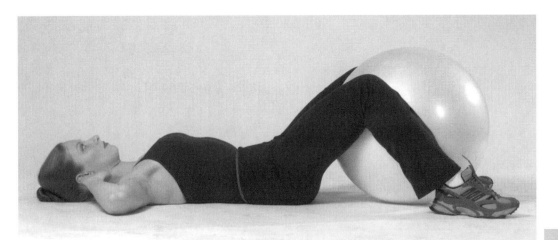

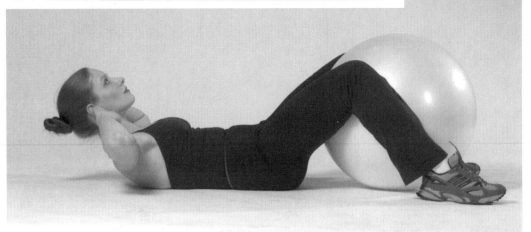

The Pike

This is a *very* advanced exercise, so be careful!

TECHNIQUE & FORM

Lie on the ball and walk your hands out until your ankles are on the ball's apex. Keeping your legs straight, draw the ball toward your hands, but do not bend your knees.

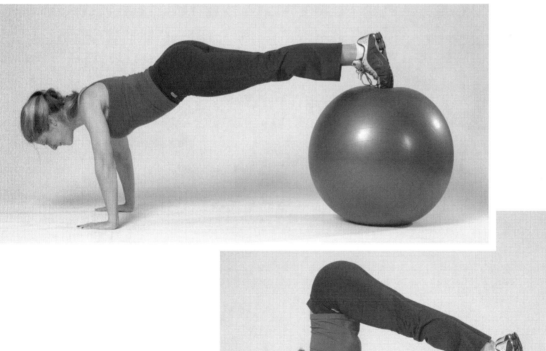

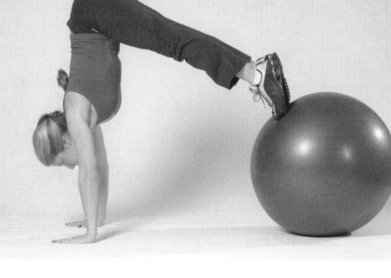

Pike Crunch

This is a *very* advanced exercise, so you will most likely have to work up to it.

TECHNIQUE & FORM
Lie on the floor with the ball between your ankles and your arms extended behind you. Simultaneously lift your shoulder blades and the ball off the floor and transfer the ball from your ankles to your hands. Return to the original position, then repeat.

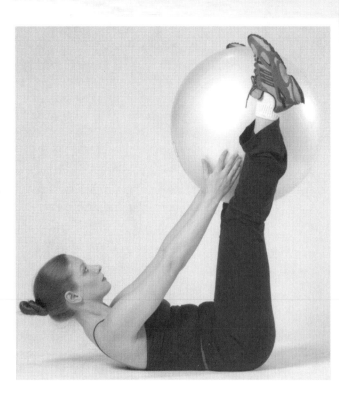

Ab Roll

The **Ab Roll** is an advanced move that will challenge both your abs and your lower back.

TECHNIQUE & FORM

Kneel in front of the ball. Place your forearms on ball's apex with your fingers interlaced. Roll the ball forward until your arms, hips, and knees are in a straight line.

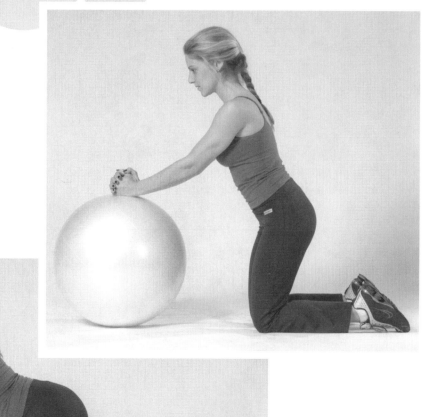

89

Scissor Rotations

This is another advanced exercise, so don't be surprised—or disappointed—if you have to work up to it.

TECHNIQUE & FORM

Lie on the floor with your hands extended and your palms on the floor. Place the ball between your ankles and squeeze. Lift your legs to a 45-degree angle, and then rotate your legs to the right as far as you can without lifting your shoulders off the floor. Repeat on the other side.

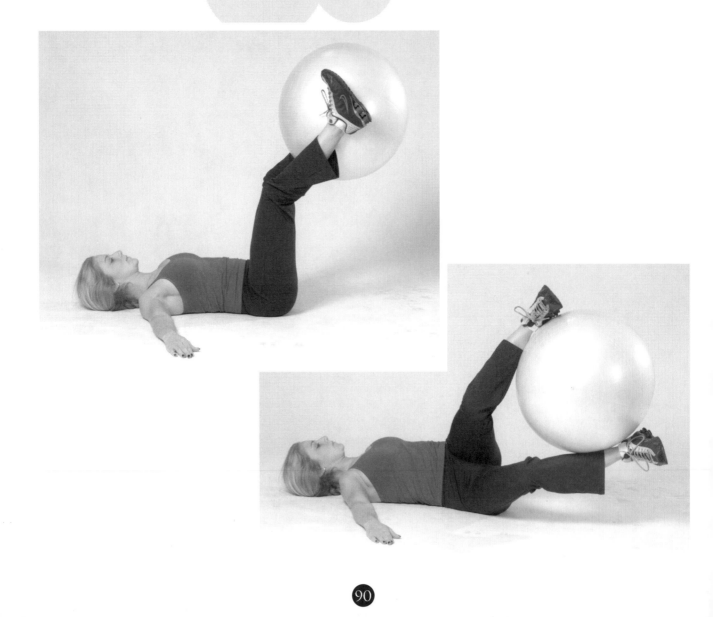

Legs

Abductors, adductors, hamstrings, quadriceps, calves

Who doesn't want long, sleek, sculpted legs? Of course, wanting them and actually having them are two entirely different matters. To get the legs of your dreams requires some work and a healthy dose of commitment on your part. The good news is that the following pages are loaded with plenty of leg blasting (and beautifying) exercises.

The Exercises

Wall Squats, page 92

Single Leg Squat, page 93

Sitting Leg Extensions, page 94

Prone Leg Extensions, page 95

Lunge & Roll, page 96

Advanced Lunge & Roll, page 97

The Lift, page 98

The Lift Variations, page 99

Hamstring Curls, page 100

Inner Thigh Flex, page 101

Single Leg Curls, page 102

Wall Squats

These are terrific for your thighs (*quadriceps, rectus femoris, vastus lateralis, vastus medialis, vastus intermedius*).

Paul's Pro Tip
Avoid locking your knees in the starting position.

TECHNIQUE & FORM

Stand in front of a wall with your feet at least shoulder width apart. Place the ball between your lower back and the wall. You should be far enough from the wall so that when you squat, your knees don't go beyond your toes. Keep your heels firmly on the ground. Slowly lower your butt to the level of your knees (the back of your thighs should be parallel to floor) and then slowly return to the starting position.

VARIATION

Hold a set of weights at your shoulders as you lower and raise yourself.

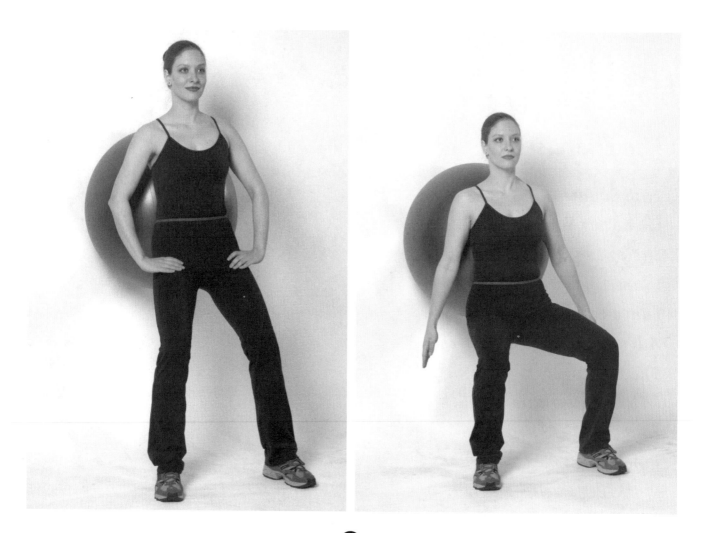

Single Leg Squat

This is an even more advanced
exercise than the *Single Leg
Stability Squat* because in
addition to lowering yourself,
you must come up again.

TECHNIQUE & FORM

Stand in front of a wall with your feet at least shoulder width
apart. Place the ball between your lower back and the wall. Lift
one foot off the floor and lower yourself until the planted thigh is
almost parallel to the floor. Slowly raise yourself again.

Sitting Leg Extensions

This is a good beginning level exercise for the butt and legs.

TECHNIQUE & FORM

Sit on the apex of the ball with an ankle weight on one leg. Lift the leg until it is parallel to the floor, but without locking the knee. Lower the leg again and repeat. Switch the weight to the opposite leg and continue.

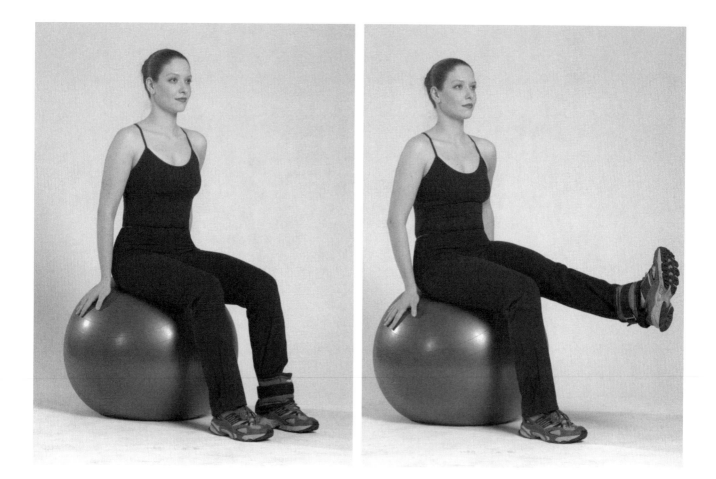

Prone Leg Extensions

TECHNIQUE & FORM

Lay on top of the ball with your hands and knees on the floor. Slowly lift one leg until it's parallel to the floor and then lower it again. Switch legs and repeat.

If you aren't able to place your knees and hands on the floor at the same time, you may need to use a smaller ball for this one.

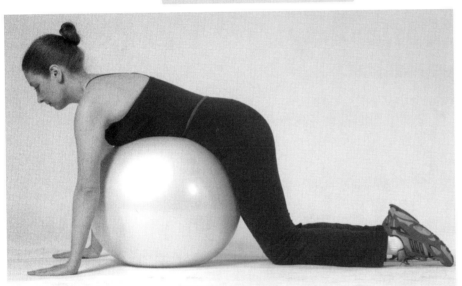

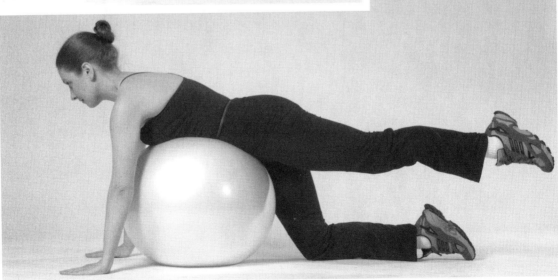

Lunge & Roll

TECHNIQUE & FORM

Stand with your feet shoulder width apart. Place your right instep on the ball behind you. Your knees should be parallel and the standing leg should be bent slightly. You can hold your hands out to the sides for more balance. Bend the standing leg and, at the same time, roll the ball backward with your foot. Lower yourself until the thigh of the lunging leg is almost parallel to the floor. As you straighten the front leg, roll the ball back to the original position.

The **Lunge & Roll** is one of the best overall exercises for the legs and glutes.

Paul's Pro Tip

When you do this exercise, you can hold your hands down by your sides or out to your sides to aid your balance. You can even brace yourself against a wall with one hand if you need to.

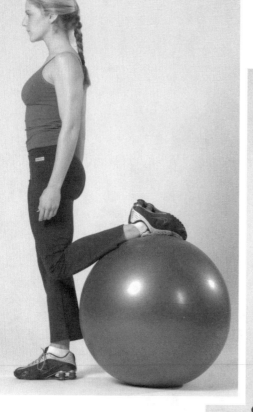

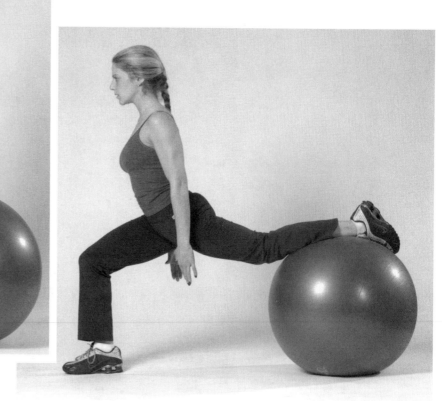

Advanced Lunge & Roll

TECHNIQUE & FORM

Start with a weight you feel comfortable lifting. Stand with your feet shoulder width apart. Place your left instep on the ball behind you. Hold the weight in your left hand. Bend the standing leg and, at the same time, roll the ball backward with your foot. At the same time, lower the weight toward the floor. Lower yourself until the thigh of the lunging leg is almost parallel to the floor. As you straighten the front leg, roll the ball back to the original position.

You may have to work up to this advanced exercise.

Paul's Pro Tip

As you lower and raise yourself, it's important to maintain the natural curve of your lower back.

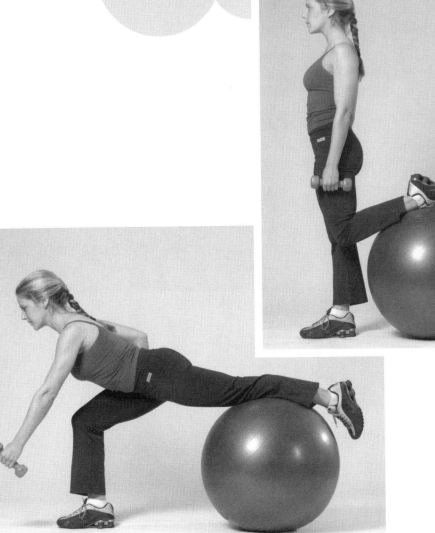

The Lift

TECHNIQUE & FORM
Lie on the ball on your hip with your legs stacked. Slowly lift and lower the top leg.

Do this exercise—which works the inner and outer thighs—and you'll discover muscles you never thought you had!

Paul's Pro Tip
Don't be surprised if the "resting" leg burns more than the lifting leg. That's because it's working overtime to keep you stable on the ball.

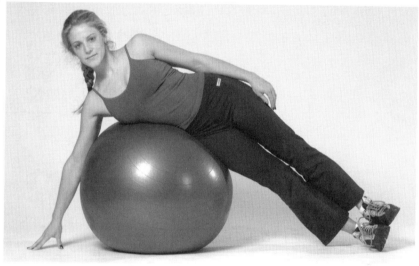

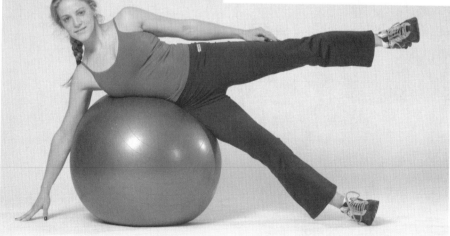

The Lift Variations

TECHNIQUE & FORM: FLEX & KICK
Lay on the ball on your hip. Flex the top knee toward your chest and extend the lower leg, keeping it parallel to the floor.

The *Flex & Kick* targets the hard-to-work outer hip.

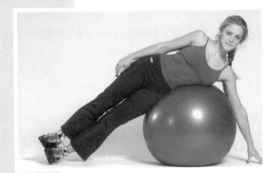

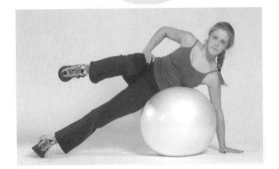 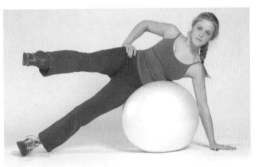

The *45-Degree Inner Thigh Flex* is a tricky exercise that will challenge your stability on the ball.

TECHNIQUE & FORM: 45-DEGREE INNER THIGH FLEX
Lie on the ball on your hip with your legs stacked. Move the top leg onto the floor and in front of the bottom leg. Bend the bottom leg at a 90-degree angle. Raise the bottom leg a few inches off the floor and then lower it again.

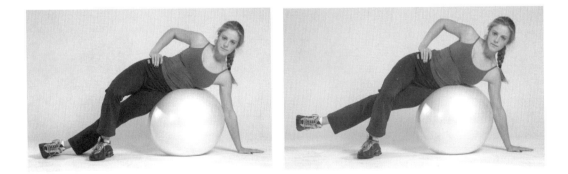

Hamstring Curls

Hamstring Curls target the muscles of your hamstrings: the *biceps femoris, semitendinosus,* and the *semimembranosus,* which most people neglect.

Paul's Pro Tip
Avoid snapping your knee joint when you do this exercise; keep your knees soft.

TECHNIQUE & FORM
Lay face up on the floor; place your ankles on top of the ball with your legs together. Keep your hips, shoulders, and head relaxed and on the floor. Extend your arms to your sides. Elevate your hips so that your ankles and shoulders are parallel, forming a straight diagonal line. Keeping your hips elevated, roll the ball in toward your butt. Roll the ball back out, and then lower your hips to the floor. Move in a smooth, controlled manner: Elevate the hips, curl in, curl out, lower the hips.

VARIATION
Changing arm positions will challenge your stability: Placing your arms at your sides is a bit more difficult. Cross them across your chest for an even more advanced variation.

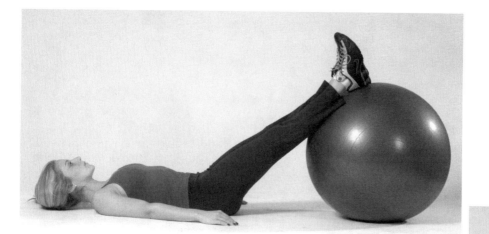

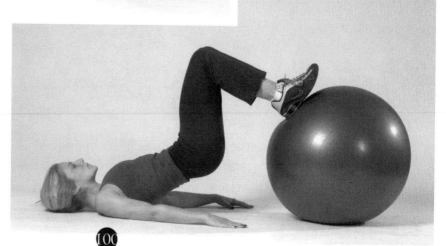

Inner Thigh Flex

TECHNIQUE & FORM
Lay on the ball on your hip with your legs stacked. Move the top leg onto the floor and in front of the bottom leg. Raise the lower leg a few inches off the floor and then lower it again.

The **Inner Thigh Flex** will help eliminate that bit of jiggle you may have around the inner thigh area.

Paul's Pro Tip
Keep the knee and toes of the lower leg facing forward at all times during the exercise. You'll have just a small range of motion, but that's okay.

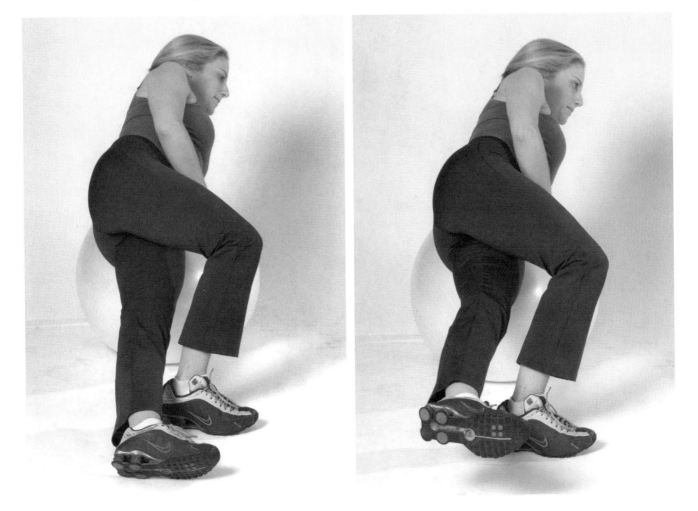

Single Leg Curls

Single Leg Curls strengthen the back of the legs, the glutes, and back. They also develop trunk and hip stability and balance.

TECHNIQUE & FORM

Lay face up on the floor with your ankles on top of the ball and your legs together. Keep your hips, shoulders, and head relaxed and on the floor. Extend your arms (with palms down) at a 90-degree angle to your sides. Lift one leg straight up off the ball. With the other leg, roll the ball in toward your butt with the other leg, and then roll it back out and place the lifted leg back on the ball. Don't drop your hips back to the floor until you've completed the set; switch legs.

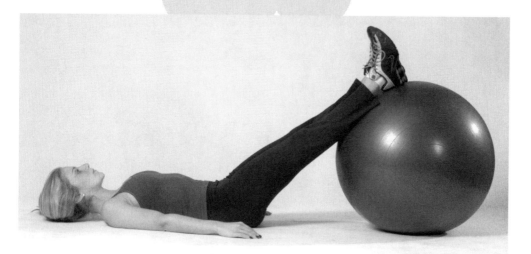

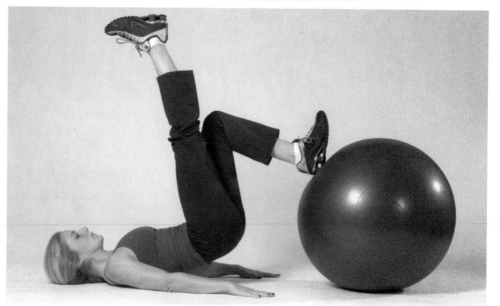

Glutes

Gluteus maximus, medius, minimus

Do you like the way you look in a pair of tight jeans? Or are you constantly shopping for baggy pants and long tops? If the latter sounds like you, fear not: The exercises in this section will carve, define, and lift your bottom.

The Exercises

Tabletop Butt Press, *page 104*

Single Leg Butt Press, *page 105*

The Twister, *page 106*

Double-Leg Extensions, *page 107*

Pulse-Ups, *page 108*

Outer Thigh Lift, *page 109*

Tabletop Butt Press

The **Tabletop Butt Press** trains the butt, the back of the legs, and lower back. It also develops trunk stability.

Paul's Pro Tip

Take care not to hyperextend in the topmost position, and modify the range of motion if you feel any lower back pain.

TECHNIQUE & FORM

Sit on the apex of the ball with your feet shoulder width apart. Slowly walk your feet forward, letting the ball roll down your back until it reaches your shoulders. Your head and neck should be comfortably resting on the ball and your butt should be close to the floor. Press your hips up so that they are parallel to your knees and then lower your hips to the ball again.

VARIATION

Place a barbell plate on your hips to increase the intensity.

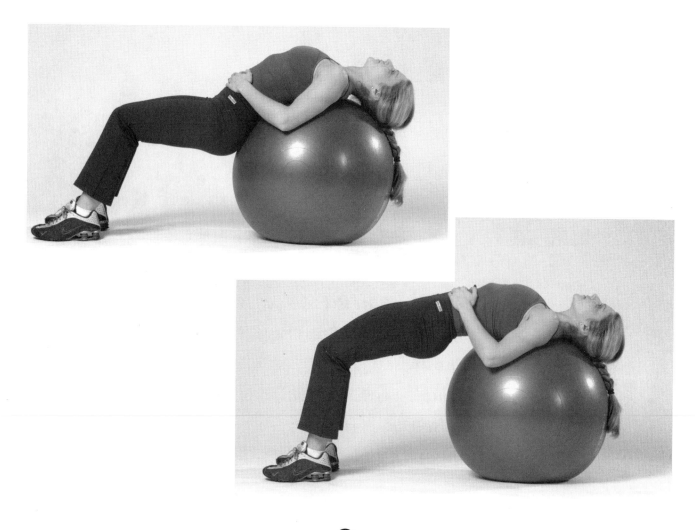

Single Leg Butt Press

The ***Single Leg Butt Press*** is an advanced and challenging exercise. It develops cross-body stability and balance.

Paul's Pro Tip

Take care not to hyperextend in the topmost position, and modify the range of motion if you feel any lower back pain.

TECHNIQUE & FORM

Sit on the apex of the ball with your feet shoulder width apart. Slowly walk your feet forward, letting the ball roll down your back until it reaches your shoulders. Your head and neck should be comfortably resting on the ball and your butt should be close to the floor. Lift one leg and extend it so that it's parallel to the floor. Stabilize yourself with the grounded foot. Keeping your hips square, press them up so that they are parallel to your knees. Slowly lower your hips back to the ball.

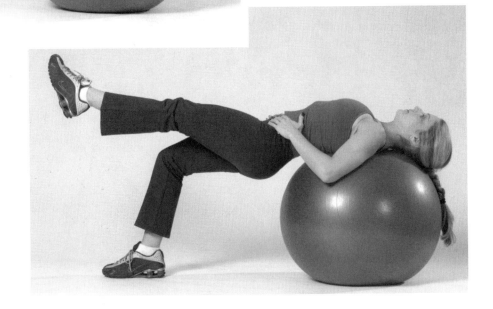

The Twister

A good deal of body control is required to do **The Twister.** It not only trains the glutes but also the waist, back, abs, and legs.

TECHNIQUE & FORM

Start with a weight that you feel comfortable lifting. Sit on the apex of the ball with your feet shoulder width apart. Slowly walk your feet forward, letting the ball roll down your back until it reaches your shoulders. Stop and elevate your hips so that they're parallel to the floor. Your head and neck should be comfortably resting on the ball. Hold the weight with both hands directly over your chest with both arms extended. With both legs firmly planted on the floor, rotate your torso to the left until the weight is parallel to the floor. Quickly change directions and then rotate to the right. Continue rotating from left to right, keeping your abdominals tight and your hips elevated.

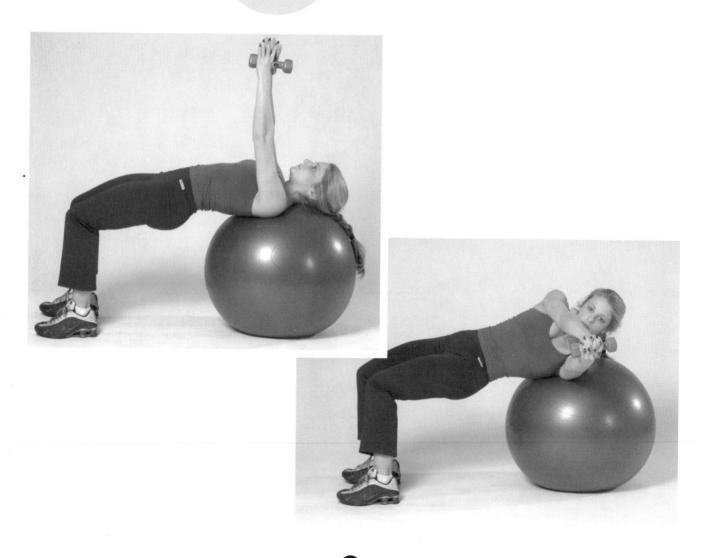

Double-Leg Extensions

TECHNIQUE & FORM
Lay on the ball with your hips on its apex. Your hands should be on the floor and your legs hip distance apart with your toes touching the floor. Do not bend your knees. Straighten your back and lift your legs until they're parallel to the floor. Hold the position for a moment, and then lower them again and repeat.

Concentrate on squeezing the gluteus muscles to lift your legs.

Paul's Pro Tip
Avoid rocking on the ball.

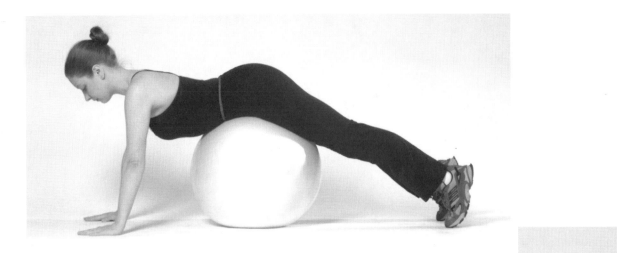

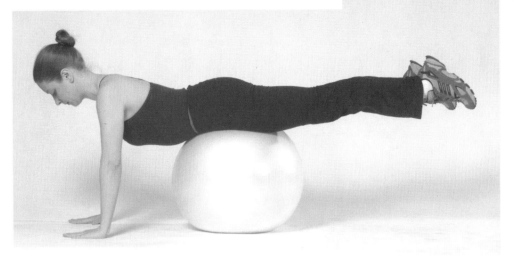

Pulse-Ups

Pulse-Ups force you to concentrate on squeezing your glutes.

Paul's Pro Tip
Avoid rocking on the ball as you perform the exercise.

TECHNIQUE & FORM
Lay on the ball with your hips on its apex. Your hands should be on the floor and your legs hip distance apart with your toes touching the floor. Lift your legs until they're parallel to the floor, and then bend your knees so that the soles of your feet are facing the ceiling. Keeping that position, pulse your legs upward. Imagine that you're pressing the soles of your feet into the ceiling. Focus on tightening the gluteus as you pulse. Don't arch your back. Pulse for the required number of reps, then slowly lower your legs to the starting position.

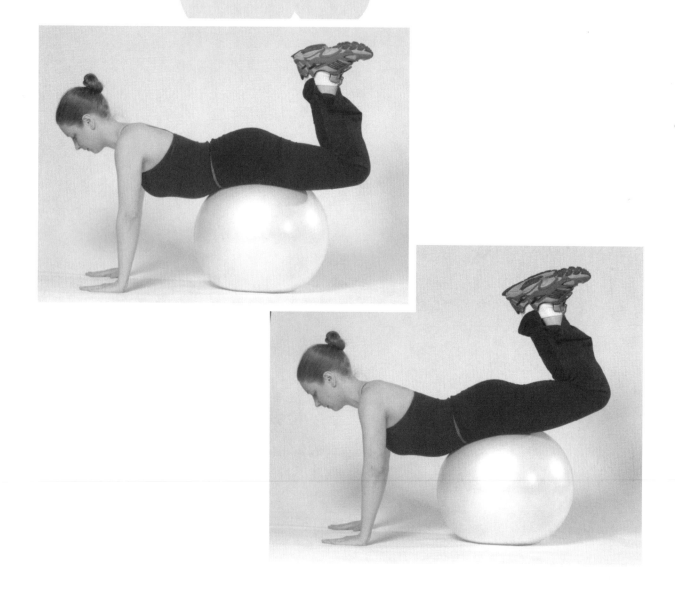

Outer Thigh Lift

TECHNIQUE & FORM
Lie on the ball on your hip with your legs stacked. Extend the top leg in front of you at a 45-degree angle. Lower and lift the leg, keeping your foot flexed.

This one's a real butt blaster!

Paul's Pro Tip
Keep the foot on the working leg flexed and the toe pointing toward the floor to keep this exercise focused on the butt.

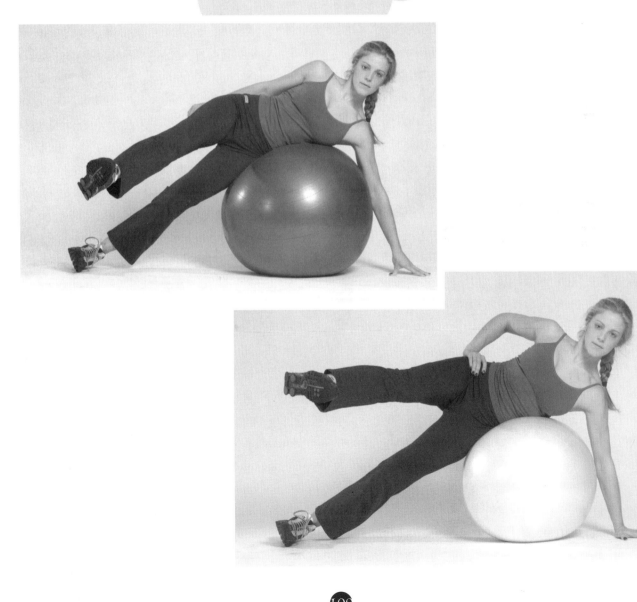

Scalenus *(anterior, medius, posterior)*
and *sternocleidomastoid*

Most of us ignore our neck muscles—that is, until we go out for a long bike ride or feel our necks burn while doing crunches in an aerobics class. These simple exercises will not only give you a lovely neck, but they'll strengthen your neck and reduce stress and neck tension.

Neck

The Exercises

Neck Extension, page 111

Neck Flexion, page 112

Lateral Neck Press, page 113

Neck Extension

The **Neck Extension** may look simple, but it really works muscles that are rarely ever worked.

TECHNIQUE & FORM

Lay face down on the ball with your chest on the ball and your feet shoulder width apart. Raise your chin off the ball until your neck is in alignment with your spine and then return to the starting position.

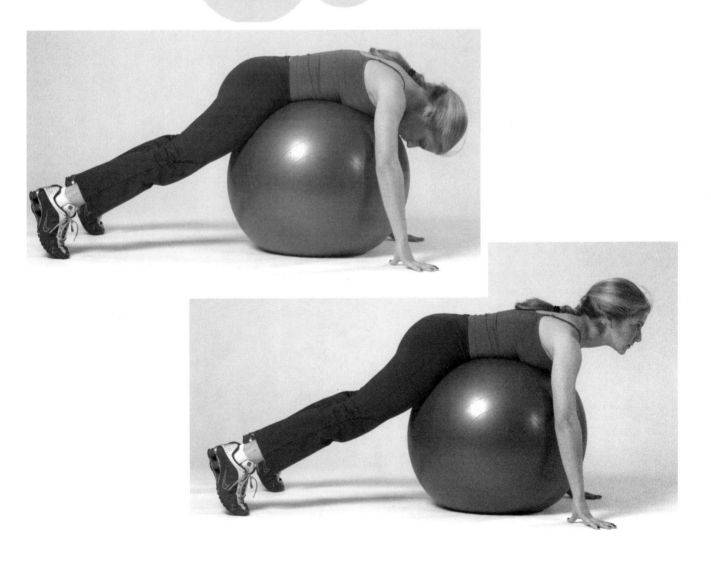

Neck Flexion

This is the exercise that will strengthen your neck so that it doesn't hurt when you do crunches.

Paul's Pro Tip
Do not do this exercise if it makes you dizzy.

TECHNIQUE & FORM
Sit on the apex of the ball, with your feet shoulder width apart. Slowly walk your feet forward, letting the ball roll down your back until it reaches your shoulders. Raise your head off the ball and then lower it to the original position.

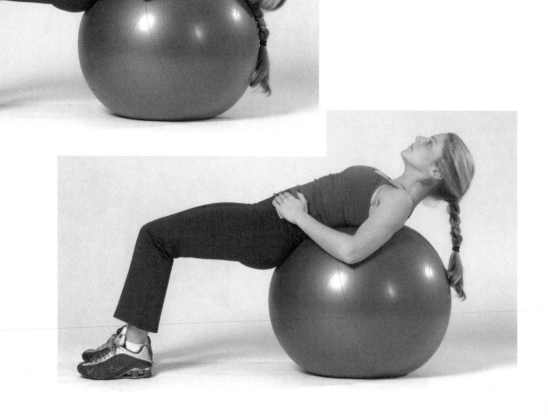

Lateral Neck Press

This one works the side of your neck—you may have never worked those!

TECHNIQUE & FORM

Place the ball against a wall. Get down on your hands and knees and place the side of your head against the ball. Press the ball against the wall with the side of your head. Hold for 3 seconds and then release. Repeat several times. Do both your left and right sides.

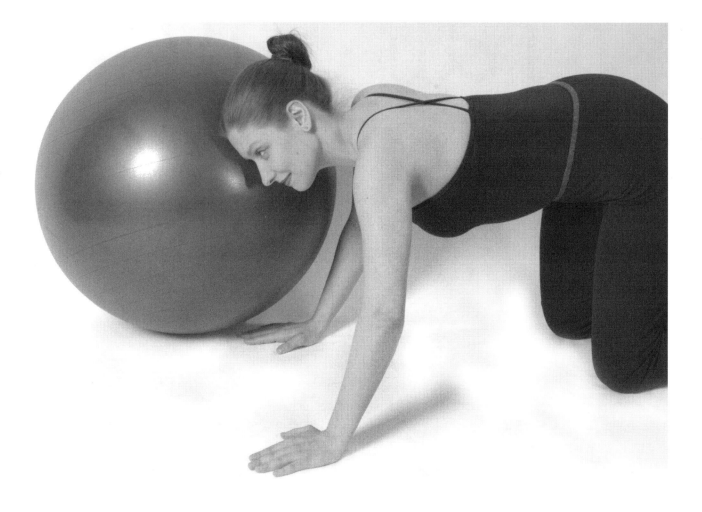

Chapter 5

PowerScu
Flexibilit
Training

If you're committed to getting and staying in shape, then you must make stretching an integral part of your exercise program. As we age, our joints and muscles naturally tighten. Stretching will slow this process. And if you stretch with consistency and diligence, you can even reverse it.

Whether you have been active in sports for years, are a fitness addict, or even if you've never exercised, you've developed muscle imbalances—imbalances that will, over time, create poor postural habits. Those in turn, create wear and tear on your joints.

Stretching a body part that you feel is tight might temporarily relieve tightness, but that tightness will return if the surrounding muscles are also tight. You know the old song that goes, "the knee bone's connected to the thigh bone"? Well, stretching, like PowerSculpt training, needs to be done in synergy—not isolation. What that means is that you need to stretch your body as a unit. Of course, you can always focus more on tight areas of your body when you stretch using a fitness ball.

There has been a slew of articles that claim stretching neither improves sports per-

lpt
y

formance nor decreases the possibility of injury. The simple reason that these claims have been made is that the conventional manner of stretching—holding a stretch for twenty-five to sixty seconds—relaxes and elongates the muscles. This "static" stretching does nothing to prepare muscles for the quick movements most sports require.

To properly prepare to work out or play sports you must warm-up and stretch in a dynamic and rhythmic fashion: Moving in and out of a stretch briskly, holding a stretch for two to three seconds and preferably using movements that are similar to your chosen activity.

Static stretching should be done after your activity or sport, when your muscles are thoroughly warmed. That's the perfect time to elongate and relax muscles. Stretching after a workout will also keep the muscles from quickly cooling off and becoming tighter than they were before the workout.

The Exercises

Shoulders, *page 116*

Chest I, *page 117*

Chest II, *page 118*

Waist, *page 119*

Back, *page 120*

Glutes, *page 121*

Quadriceps, *page 122*

Hamstrings, *page 123*

Shoulders

TECHNIQUE & FORM

Kneel in front of, and then place both hands on top of the ball. Roll the ball forward (your chest will move toward the floor). Then roll the ball to the left and the right to stretch different muscle fibers.

Paul's Pro Tip

Pay attention to your breathing as you perform this and every other stretch in this section. People often hold their breath as they stretch.

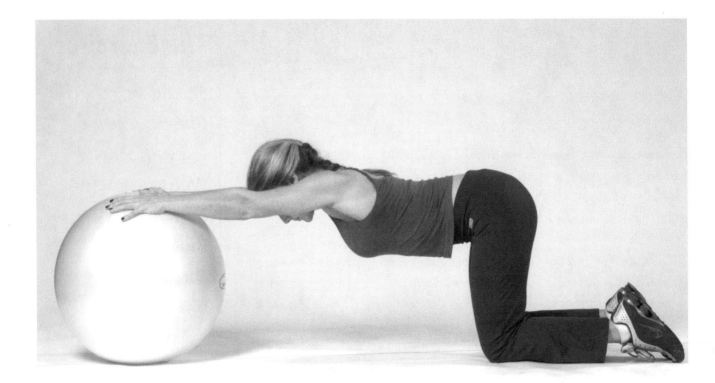

Chest I

TECHNIQUE & FORM

Kneel on the floor with the ball on your right side. Place your right hand on top of the ball. Roll the ball backward and move your body forward so that your chest draws toward the floor. Hold 2 to 3 seconds and repeat. Repeat on both sides.

Paul's Pro Tip

You can avoid stress on your wrists while doing this stretch by keeping your fingers spread wide and distributing your weight throughout your hands and fingers.

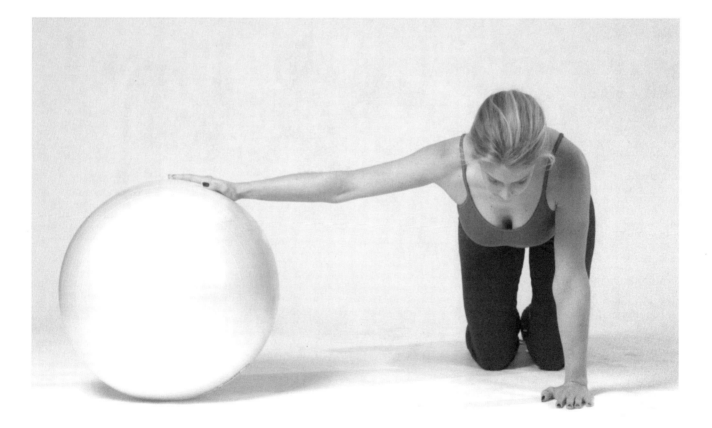

Chest II

TECHNIQUE & FORM

Sit on the apex of the ball, and then walk forward until the ball is supporting your lower back. Stretch out your arms to the sides. Hold 2 to 3 seconds and repeat.

Besides relieving daily fatigue, this stretch is great to do in the morning to relieve nighttime stiffness. It stretches and opens your chest.

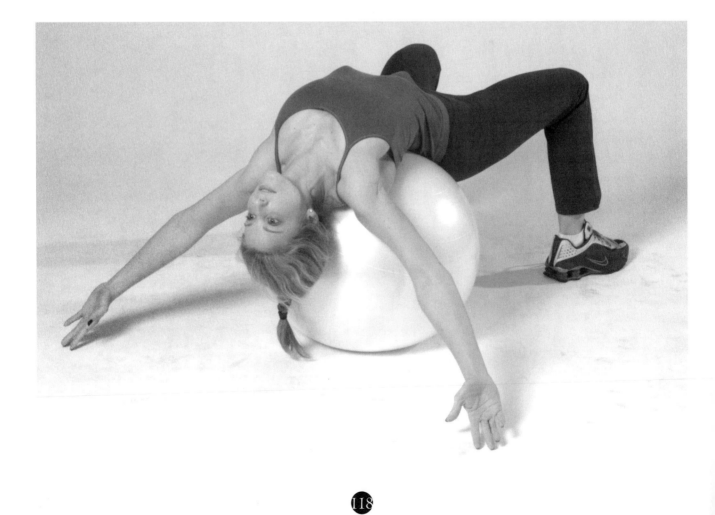

Waist

This stretch is essential after any abdominal training.

Paul's Pro Tip
Changing your arm position can increase the stretch.

TECHNIQUE & FORM

Sit on the apex of the ball, and then walk your feet forward until you're lying on top of the ball. This position stretches the **rectus abdominis**, the long sheet of muscle that runs down the middle of your abdomen. Hold 2 to 3 seconds. From this position, rotate to one side and reach the top arm over your head. Keep your feet wide apart for balance. Hold 2 to 3 seconds. This segment of the position stretches your waist.

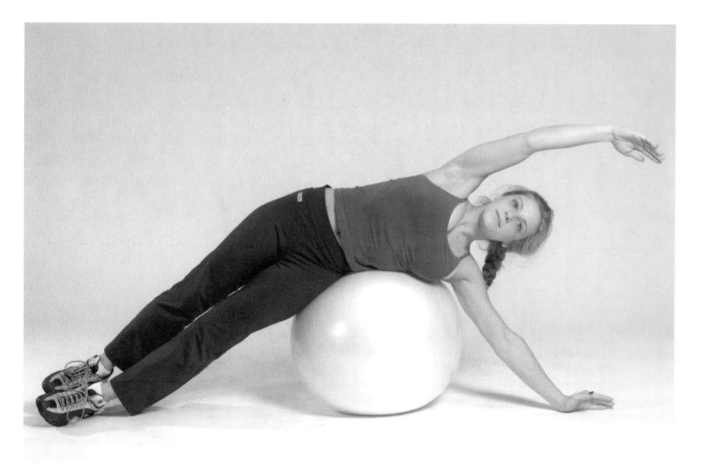

Back

Breathe deeply as you perform this stretch and you'll feel your range of motion gently increasing.

TECHNIQUE & FORM

Sit on the apex of the ball with your feet wide apart and flat on the floor. Lower your head between your knees and reach your hands toward the floor. Keep your neck and shoulders relaxed. Hold 2 to 3 seconds and repeat.

VARIATION

For a deeper stretch, wrap your arms around the inside of your calves.

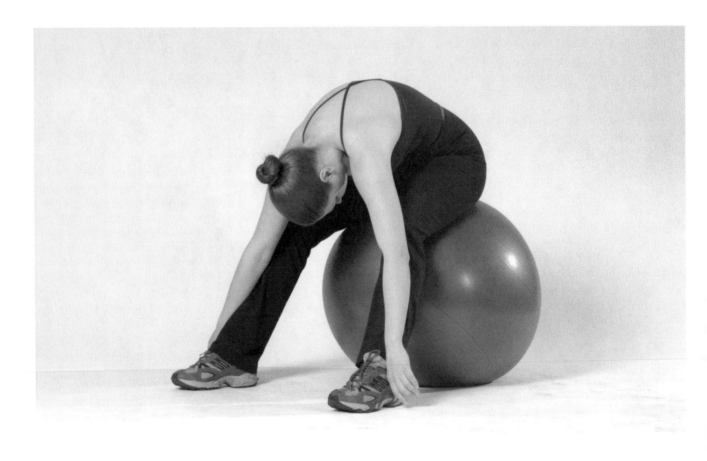

Glutes

This stretch is related to the pigeon pose in yoga. It not only stretches the glutes, but also opens the hips.

TECHNIQUE & FORM
Place the lateral side of your bent knee on the top of the ball with the opposite leg extended behind you. Place both hands on the ball in front of you (as you become more flexible, drop your hands toward the floor in front of you), while bringing your chest toward the bent knee. Roll the ball around to target different muscle fibers.

Front view

Quadriceps

TECHNIQUE & FORM
Place one knee on the floor, then place the instep of that foot on the ball. Hold 2 to 3 seconds and repeat. You'll feel the stretch in the front of your thigh.

Paul's Pro Tip
To increase this stretch and stretch the hip flexor, press your hips away from the ball.

If you're less flexible, use a smaller ball. If you're more flexible, a larger ball is more suitable.

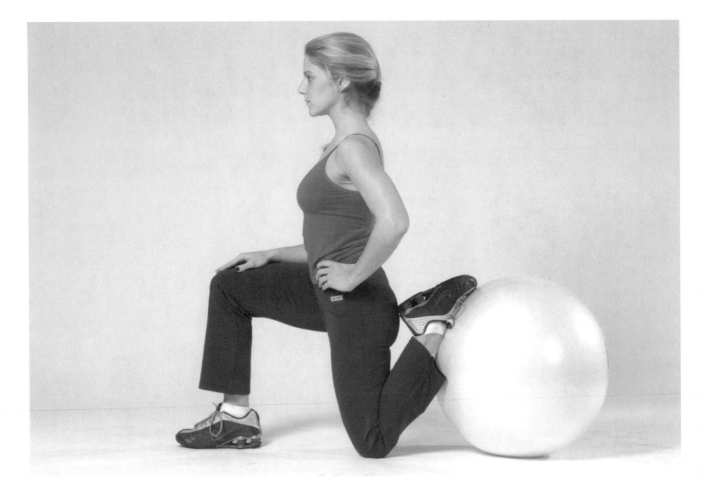

Hamstrings

Paul's Pro Tip
Don't slouch as you perform this stretch; keep your back as straight as possible.

TECHNIQUE & FORM
Sit on the apex of the ball with your knees bent at a 90-degree angle and your feet flat on the floor. Push back on your heels, straighten your legs, and pull your toes toward your shins. Hold 2 to 3 seconds and repeat.

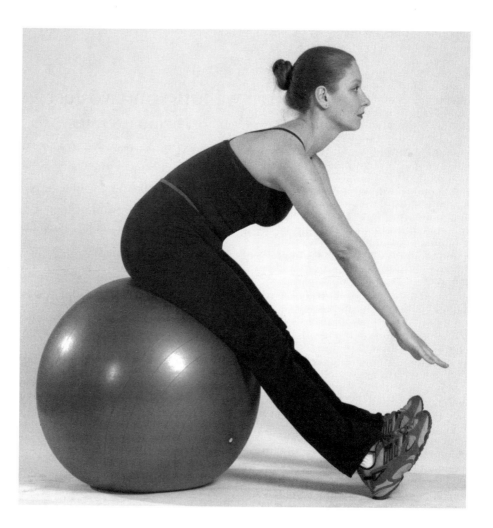

Chapter 6

PowerSculpt Balance

If you're walking on two feet you have at least some balance. Most individuals refuse to do any balance training because they think it's not important. It can also seem to be very tedious, boring, and quite frankly a waste of time. So why is balance important, anyway? If you participate in active pursuits that require coordination, agility, or quick footwork—think biking, hiking, ice skating, in-line skating, skiing, or windsurfing—balance training will improve your performance. Balance conditioning improves your posture. When you have good balance, you waste less energy and move more efficiently.

Even if you're not into traditional sports, you probably still walk down stairs, carry heavy loads occasionally, run for the bus, or reach for something on a high shelf. Good balance will help you with all those day-to-day tasks, too. Here's a quick way to test your balance: See how long you can stand on one foot while keeping your other leg bent. Handle that pretty well? Now do the same thing with your eyes closed. It might not be so easy.

The fitness ball is a wonderful tool for enhancing balance. Almost any exercise you do on it challenges your balance, but the poses on the following pages are especially effective for testing—and improving your balance.

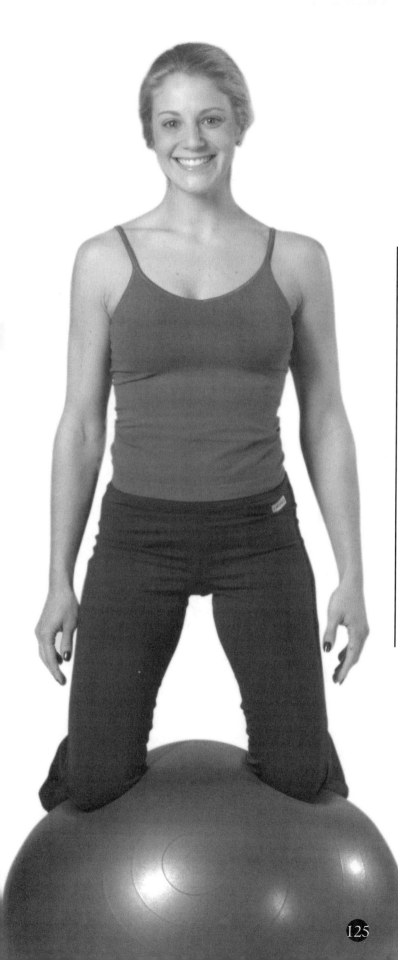

The Exercises

Sitting on the Ball, page 126

Sitting with One Foot Elevated, page 127

Sitting with One Leg Extended, page 128

Two-Point Perch, page 129

Three-Point Perch, page 130

Four-Point Perch, page 131

The Pose, page 132

Two-Point Cross Stance, page 133

Sitting on the Ball

Sitting on the Ball is the first step in practicing balance.

TECHNIQUE & FORM
Sit upright on the apex of the ball with your chest high and your shoulders back.

VARIATION
Move your arms to different positions and see how your body compensates to maintain your balance.

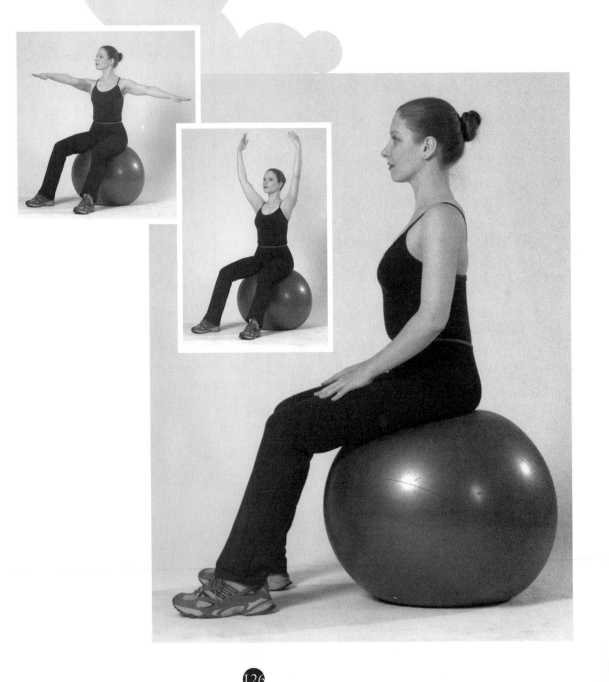

Sitting with One Foot Elevated

It may look simple, but don't be surprised if you have a hard time at first.

TECHNIQUE & FORM

Sit upright on the apex of the ball. Lift one foot a couple of inches off the floor. Change your arm position and try to maintain your balance. Switch legs and repeat.

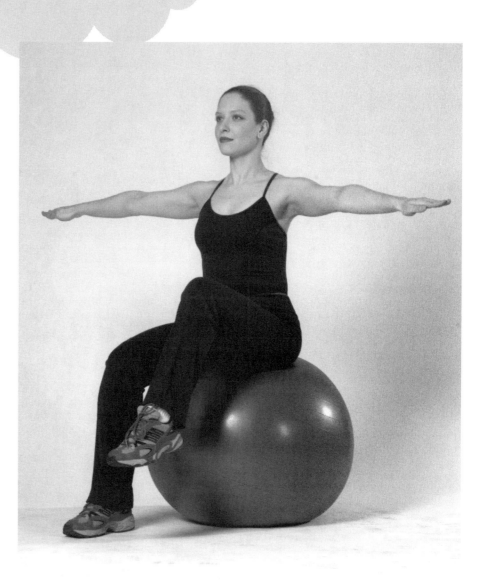

Sitting with One Leg Extended

TECHNIQUE & FORM
Sit upright on the apex of the ball. Lift one foot off the floor and then extend the leg until it's parallel to the floor. Change your arm position and try to maintain your balance.

You may find it easiest to maintain this position with your arms extended out to your sides.

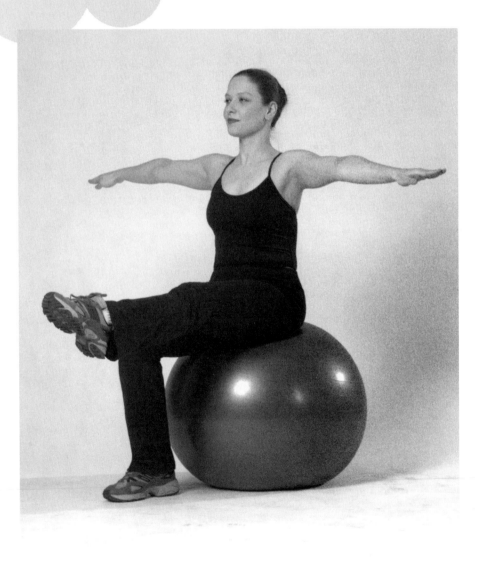

Two-Point Perch

TECHNIQUE & FORM
From the Four-Point Perch position, lift both hands off the ball.

As you do this pose, feel how much your hips and glutes need to work to stabilize your body in this position. Feel free to brace yourself against a wall until you're able to balance on your own.

Paul's Pro Tip
Once you're comfortable in this position, play catch with a partner using a tennis ball.

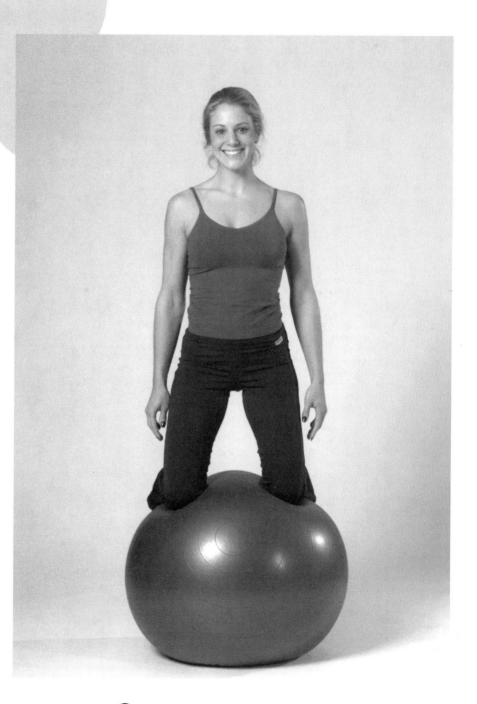

Variation: Three-Point Perch

TECHNIQUE & FORM

From the Four-Point Perch position lift one hand off the ball and extend the arm in front of you. Switch arms and repeat.

Paul's Pro Tip

Lift your arm slowly off the ball. Keeping your eyes focused on an object in front of you will help you keep your balance.

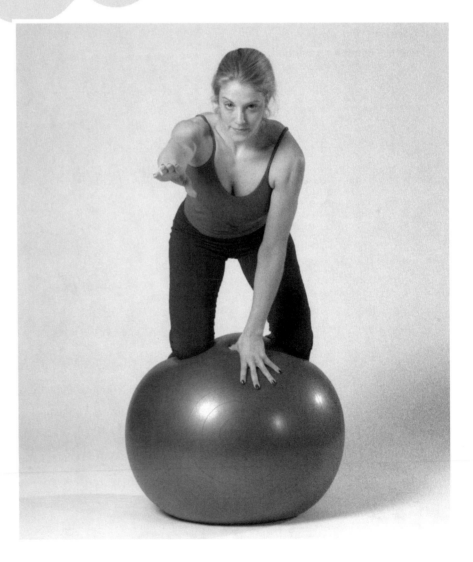

Variation: Four-Point Perch

TECHNIQUE & FORM
Stand in front of the ball. Place your hands on top and then gently allow your weight to roll you forward until your hands and knees are on the ball.

Build up to holding this pose for one to two minutes.

Paul's Pro Tip
Keeping your insteps on the ball will give you better control. Until you're able to execute this pose, support yourself against a wall with two and then one hand.

The Pose

TECHNIQUE & FORM

Start in the Four-Point Perch position. Lift the sole of one foot onto the ball while stabilizing yourself with your hands and the opposite knee. Once you're comfortable, lift both hands off the ball.

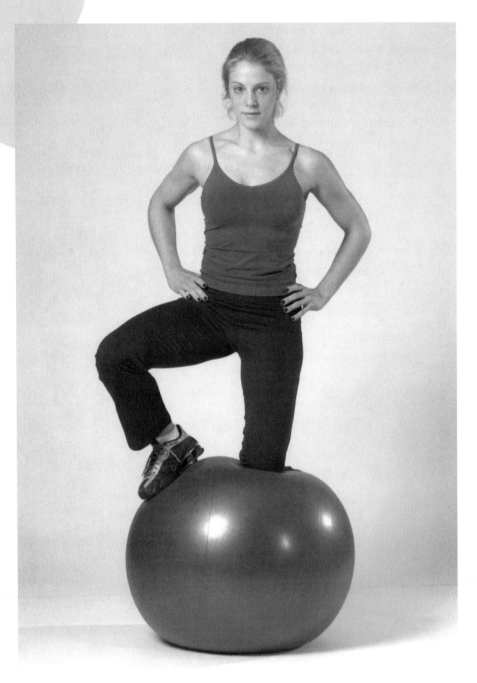

Two-Point Cross Stance

TECHNIQUE & FORM
While in the Four-Point Perch position, extend one arm and the opposite leg. Switch and repeat.

This pose requires strong cross-body stabilization. It's not unusual to be strong on one side and weak on the other.

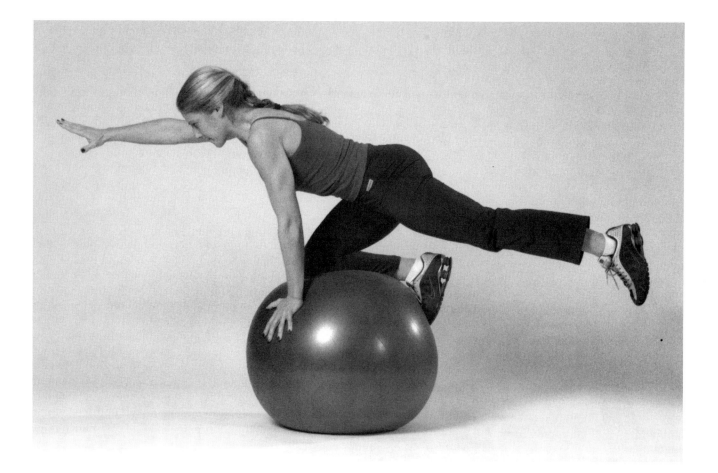

Chapter 7

The PowerSculpt Workouts

Following the PowerSculpt Workouts sequentially —starting with Stage I—is essential for developing a safe, effective, progressive, and successful training regimen. Here are some general points to keep in mind: No two individuals are alike. The number of reps and sets are general recommendations. The workouts should be challenging—not impossible. And never, ever sacrifice form to complete a set.

Stage 1: Stability & Foundations

•Do three workouts per week for three weeks.

•If you find you're not able to progress to Stage 2 after three weeks, simply repeat Stage I.

This stage is for anyone new to fitness ball training, beginner exercisers, or seniors. But keep in mind that these Stage 1 exercises can be used as a workout, a warm-up, a balance primer, and a stretch program. You're ready to move to Stage 2 when you: (1) can hold the Stability poses for the time alloted for beginners; (2) can complete all the Warm-Ups and Balance poses; and (3) have charted your range of motion for the Stretches.

Stability

Stability Moves
start on page 18.

- Time: 10 minutes.
- Do each of the Stability moves and keep track of the time you're able to hold each position.
- If you aren't able to hold the position for the time allotted for Beginners, rest and repeat the exercise until you've made up the time. For example, if you can hold the Shoulder Girdle Protraction pose for only 5 seconds, rest for 1 minute and then repeat the exercise for 4 sets of 5 seconds each.

Warm-Up

Warm-Ups
start on page 26.

- Time: 10 minutes.
- Do all the Warm-Up exercises in a pain-free range of motion.
- Start the movements slowly and pay attention to your posture.
- Avoid any warm-ups that feel uncomfortable or that make you feel dizzy.
- Start by doing 5 to 10 of each.

Balance

Balance Moves
start on page 124.

- Time: 3 to 5 minutes.
- Choose a level with which you're comfortable—I recommend starting with the sitting balance exercises, which are challenging despite the fact that you're sitting.
- One note: You may discover that you can do these exercises well on one day but have trouble on another day. Don't worry...that's quite normal.

Stretching

Stretches
start on page 114.

- Time: 10 to 20 minutes.
- Perform all of the stretches you can while staying in a pain-free range of motion. Chart your progress.

PowerSculpt Stage 2: Adaptation

In Stage 2 your body will begin to adapt to training with weights on the fitness ball. You will strengthen muscles, tendons, and ligaments in preparation for more advanced levels.

For the weight-training, choose a weight that's heavy enough for you to just complete the number of reps called for, but not so heavy that it alters your form. You should be challenged—not strained.

• Do three workouts per week for three weeks.

• Begin each workout with a 10-minute warm-up.

• Finish with 10 minutes of stretching.

Chest

Week 1	Week 2	Week 3
12 Hands-on-Floor Push-Ups	15 Hands-on-Floor Push-Ups	20 Hands-on-Floor Push-Ups
12 Long Head Presses	15 Long Head Presses	20 Long Head Presses
12 Dumbbell Flies	15 Dumbbell Flies	20 Dumbbell Flies

Legs

Week 1	Week 2	Week 3
2 x 10 Squat & Press	3 x 12 Squat & Press	3 x 15 Squat & Press
2 x 10 Hamstring Curls	3 x 12 Hamstring Curls	3 x 15 Hamstring Curls

Arms/Back/Shoulders

Week 1	Week 2	Week 3
10 One-Arm Standing Rows	12 One-Arm Standing Rows	15 One-Arm Standing Rows
10 Back Extensions	12 Back Extensions	15 Back Extensions
10 Prone Rows	12 Prone Rows	15 Prone Rows
3 x 10 Biceps Combo[1]	3 x 12 Biceps Combo[1]	3 x 15 Biceps Combo[1]
3 x 10 Triceps Combo[2]	3 x 10 Triceps Combo[2]	3 x 10 Triceps Combo[2]

[1] 1 set of Seated Biceps Curls, 1 set of Tabletop Biceps Curls, 1 set of Preacher Curls.

[2] 1 set of Standing Triceps Extensions, 1 set of Seated Overhead Extensions, 1 set of Tabletop Triceps Extensions.

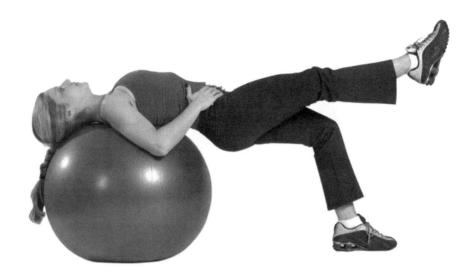

Abs

Week 1	Week 2	Week 3
25 Crunches	30 Crunches	35 Crunches
25 Reverse Crunches	30 Reverse Crunches	35 Reverse Crunches
25 Crunches w/Rotation	30 Crunches w/Rotation	35 Crunches w/Rotation

Balance

Choose 1 balance exercise and practice for
2 minutes on each of the three days.

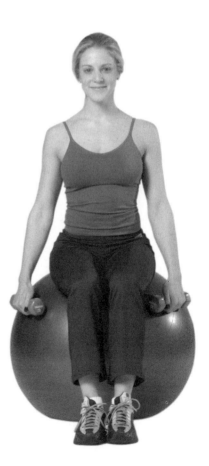

PowerSculpt Stage 3: Strength

In Stage 3 you'll get stronger by decreasing the number of reps you do and increaing the amount of weight or intensity of the exercise. But don't worry about building huge, unattractive muscles—it's simply much more difficult for women to get "bulked up" than it is for men. What building muscles does is increase your body's ability to burn fat.

- Do three workouts per week for three weeks.
- Begin each workout with a 10-minute warm-up
- Finish with 10 minutes of stretching

Chest

Week 1	Week 2	Week 3
15 Hands-on-Floor Push-Ups	12 Hands-on-Floor Push-Ups	10 Hands-on-Floor Push-Ups
15 Long Head Presses	12 Long Head Presses	10 Long Head Presses
15 Dumbbell Flies	12 Dumbbell Flies	10 Dumbbell Flies

Legs

Week 1	Week 2	Week 3
3 x 15 Squat & Press	3 x 12 Squat & Press	3 x 10 Squat & Press
3 x 15 Hamstring Curls	3 x 12 Hamstring Curls	3 x 12 Hamstring Curls

Back

Week 1	Week 2	Week 3
10 One-Arm Standing Rows	12 One-Arm Standing Rows	15 One-Arm Standing Rows
10 Back Extensions	12 Back Extensions	15 Back Extensions
10 Prone Rows	12 Prone Rows	15 Prone Rows

Shoulders

Week 1	Week 2	Week 3
1 x 15 Seated Lateral Raises	1 x 12 Seated Lateral Raises	1 x 10 Seated Lateral Raises
1 x 15 Anterior Raises	1 x 12 Anterior Raises	1 x 10 Seated Posterior Extensions
1 x 15 Seated Posterior Extensions	1 x 12 Seated Lateral Raises	1 x 10 Seated Lateral Raises

For the weight-training, choose a weight that's heavy enough for you to just complete the number of reps called for, but not so heavy that it alters your form. You should be challenged—not strained. If you find your form or posture is breaking down, grab a lighter weight.

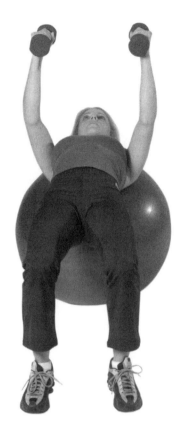

Hips/Butt/Thighs

Week 1	Week 2	Week 3
1 x 15 Tabletop Butt Presses	1 x 12 Lifts	1 x 10 Lifts
1 x 15 Inner Thigh Flexes	1 x 12 Inner Thigh Flexes	1 x 10 Tabletop Butt Presses
1 x 15 Lifts	1 x 12 Tabletop Butt Presses	1 x 10 Lifts

Arms

Week 1	Week 2	Week 3
3 x 10 Biceps Combo[1]	3 x 12 Biceps Combo[1]	3 x 15 Biceps Combo[1]
3 x 10 Triceps Combo[2]	3 x 10 Triceps Combo[2]	3 x 10 Triceps Combo[2]

[1] 1 set of Seated Biceps Curls, 1 set of Tabletop Biceps Curls, 1 set of Preacher Curls.

[2] 1 set of Standing Triceps Extensions, 1 set of Seated Overhead Extensions, 1 set of Tabletop Triceps Extensions.

Abs

Week 1	Week 2	Week 3
25 Crunches	30 Crunches	35 Crunches
25 Reverse Crunches	30 Reverse Crunches	35 Reverse Crunches
25 Crunches w/Rotation	30 Crunches w/Rotation	35 Crunches w/Rotation

Balance

Choose 1 balance exercise and practice it for 2 minutes on each of the three days.

PowerSculpt Stage 4: Power

Stage Four is designed for power. In this stage we will maintain the intensity of weight as in Stage 2, but vary the speed in three levels:

Fast (as fast as you can do the exercise without losing form)

Medium (a standard 3 count up and 3 count down)

Slow (count 10 up and 10 down) when you do the exercises.

• Do three workouts per week for 3 weeks.

• Alternate and vary the speed of each set. Stage Four is a 3-week, 3 times per week program.

• Begin each workout with a 10-minute warm-up.

• Finish with 10 minutes of stretching.

Chest

Week 1	Week 2	Week 3
15 Hands-on-Floor Push-Ups	12 Hands-on-Floor Push-Ups	10 Hands-on-Floor Push-Ups
15 Long Head Presses	12 Long Head Presses	10 Long Head Presses
15 Dumbbell Flies	12 Dumbbell Flies	10 Dumbbell Flies

Legs

Week 1	Week 2	Week 3
2 x 15 Wall Squats	1 x 12 Wall Squats	1 x 10 Wall Squats
2 x 15 Hamstring Curls	2 x 12 Hamstring Curls	2 x 12 Hamstring Curls
1 x 15 Single Leg Squats	2 x 12 Single Leg Squats	3 x 10 Single Leg Squats

Back

Week 1	Week 2	Week 3
15 One-Arm Standing Rows	12 One-Arm Standing Rows	10 One-Arm Standing Rows
15 Back Extensions	12 Back Extensions	10 Back Extensions
15 Prone Rows	12 Prone Rows	10 Prone Rows

Shoulders

Week 1	Week 2	Week 3
1 x 15 Seated Lateral Raises	1 x 12 Seated Posterior Extensions	1 x 10 Anterior Raises
1 x 15 Anterior Raises	1 x 12 Anterior Raises	1 x 10 Seated Posterior Extensions
1 x 15 Seated Posterior Extensions	1 x 12 Seated Lateral Raises	1 x 10 Seated Lateral Raises

Hips/Butt/Thighs

Week 1	Week 2	Week 3
1 x 15 Tabletop Butt Presses	1 x 12 Lifts	1 x 10 Inner Thigh Lifts
1 x 15 Inner Thigh Lifts	1 x 12 Inner Thigh Lifts	1 x 10 Table Top Butt Presses
1 x 15 Lifts	1 x 12 Tabletop Butt Presses	1 x 10 Lifts

Biceps/Triceps

Week 1	Week 2	Week 3
3 x 15 Biceps Combo[1]	3 x 12 Biceps Combo[1]	3 x 10 Biceps Combo[1]
3 x 15 Triceps Combo[2]	3 x 12 Triceps Combo[2]	3 x 10 Triceps Combo[2]

[a] 1 set of seated Biceps Curls, 1 set of Half Tabletop Biceps Curls, 1 set of Kneeling Biceps Curls.

[b] 1 set of Overhead Triceps , 1 set of Triceps Extensions, 1 set of Seated TK.

Abs

Week 1	Week 2	Week 3
25 Crunches	30 Crunches	35 Crunches
25 Reverse Crunches	30 Reverse Crunches	35 Reverse Crunches
25 Crunches w/Rotation	30 Crunches w/Rotation	35 Crunches w/Rotation

Balance

Choose a balance exercise and practice for 2 minutes.

PowerSculpt Blast Circuit

The PowerSculpt Blast Circuit is an intensive body sculpting program. You'll work out one day a week for ten weeks.

The PowerSculpt Blast Circuit pushes a chosen muscle group as far as it can go, then lets it recover for six full days. With warm-up and stretch, each workout will last anywhere from 30 to 45 minutes.

- Begin with a 10-minute warmup.
- Choose a level in which you can complete 15 repetitions. For each consecutive set, drop the weight or intensity to a level in which you can complete the set.
- Rest 15 to 30 seconds between exercises.
- Rest 1 minute between sets.
- Complete 3 sets.
- Increase the amount of weight or intensity by 5 percent each week and decrease the number of reps by one each week.
- At the end of 5 weeks you should have increased the amount of weight you're using by 25 percent and completing 10 reps of each exercise.
- Begin weeks 6 through 10 cycle by lifting 15 percent less than what you were lifing at the end of week 5.
- Do 10 minutes of stretching after completing all 3 sets.

Chest Blast

10 to 15 Hands-on-Floor Push-Ups

10 to 15 Dumbbell Flies

10 to 15 Long Head Presses

10 to 15 Hands-on-Ball Push-Ups

10 to 15 Push & Press

Rest 10 to 15 seconds between exercises, rest 1 minute between sets. Do 3 sets.

Shoulder Blast

10 to 15 Seated Lateral Raises

10 to 15 Anterior Raises

10 to 15 Seated Posterior Raises

Rest 10 to 15 seconds between exercises, rest 1 minute between sets. Do 3 sets.

Back Blast

10 to 15 One-Arm Standing Rows

10 to 15 Back Extensions

Back Extension (hold in up position for 60 seconds)

10 to 15 Prone Rows

Rest 10 to 15 seconds between exercises, rest 1 minute between sets. Do 3 sets.

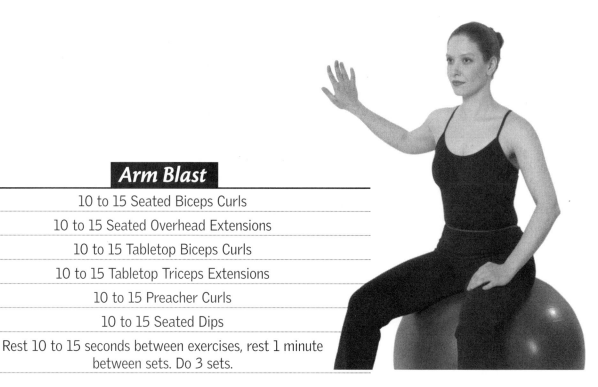

Arm Blast

10 to 15 Seated Biceps Curls

10 to 15 Seated Overhead Extensions

10 to 15 Tabletop Biceps Curls

10 to 15 Tabletop Triceps Extensions

10 to 15 Preacher Curls

10 to 15 Seated Dips

Rest 10 to 15 seconds between exercises, rest 1 minute between sets. Do 3 sets.

Hips, Buns and Thigh Blast

10 to 15 Single Leg Squats

10 to 15 Wall Squats

10 to 15 Hamstring Curls

10 to 15 Inner Thigh Flexes

10 to 15 Pulse-Ups

10 to 15 Double-Leg Extensions

Rest 10 to 15 seconds between exercises, rest 1 minute between sets. Do 3 sets.

Abs Blast

15 to 25 Crunches

15 to 25 Body Crunches

15 to 25 Reverse Crunches

15 to 25 Crunches with Rotation

15 to 25 Crunches with Knee Side Curl

60 second hold on the "up" position of the back extension
Rest 1 minute between sets. Do 3 sets.